SIT N FIT CHAIR YOGA

SIMPLE CHAIR YOGA

By KRISTINE LEE

SIT N FIT CHAIR YOGA
Simple Chair Yoga

Not all yoga postures or exercises are suitable for everyone and this or any other program may result in injury. To reduce the risk of injury, consult your doctor before beginning this or any other exercise program. The instructions and suggestions in this book are in no way intended as a substitute for medical consultation or counseling. The creators, producers and distributors of this book and program disclaim any liability or loss in connection with the exercises or advice herein.

Photographer: James Greene
Graphic Designer: Janette Robbins

ISBN 978-0-9908022-0-4
BISAC: Health & Fitness/Yoga
Second Print Edition (Color) July 2015

Printed in the United States of America

Dedication

To my family. Thank you for all your love and support on this journey.

To students, seniors, sages and teachers.

May this simple practice help you:

- *Let go of regret of the past and fear of the future*
- *Connect your quiet, compassionate mind to your miraculous body*
- *Feel the infinite peace and love that reside within*

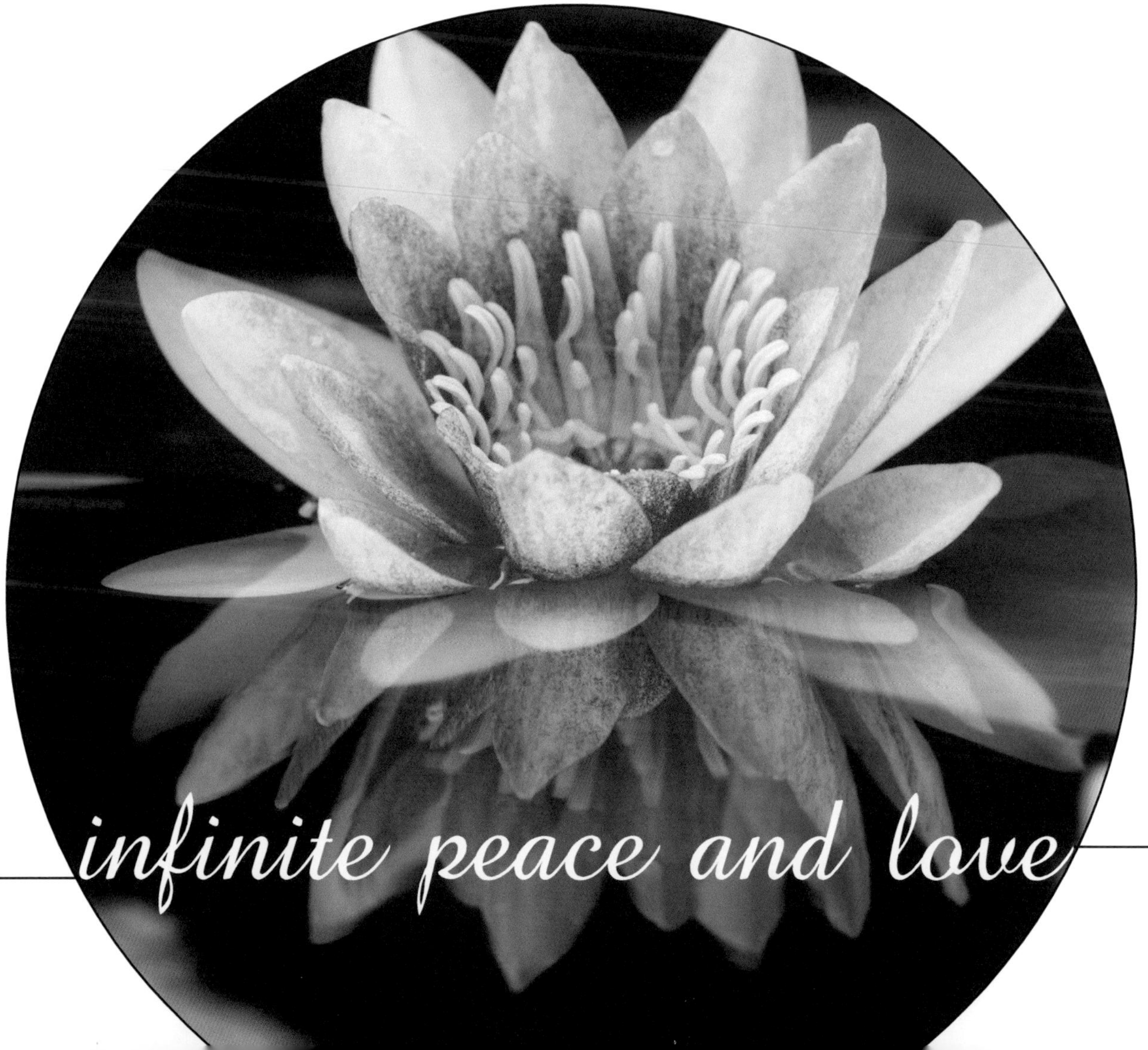

Table of Contents

Acknowledgments

I gratefully acknowledge the following for their contributions to this work.

My deep appreciation to Ron Smith, author of *The Knowledge Catcher*, and Life Coach, who encouraged me to organize my chair yoga expertise and passion into a format that is recognized as powerful and simple. Ron's contagious positive energy, zeal for life and excellence, gave me confidence and vision.

I acknowledge and thank Reverend Nancy Norman, Senior Minister and CEO of Unity of Delray Beach, who continuously inspires me and has supported me on this journey.

My sincere thanks to my yoga teachers for sharing their knowledge, wisdom, compassion, and love of yoga and people. My primary yoga teachers include: Roberta Case, Marilyn McElveen, Prem Shakti, and Joann Evans. A very special thanks to my Sit N Fit Chair Yoga teachers: Diane Zantop, Ileana Claffey, Sabah Saoud, Dotty Zevin, and Christine Apter. Your dedication and devotion to yoga is changing the world.

I gratefully thank Louise Mirkin, my devoted friend, and yoga student who took the time and patience to edit Sit N Fit Chair Yoga. A special thanks also to graphic designer, Janette Robbins, for her excellent, meticulous work and to my talented photographer, James Greene, for helping me get just the right photos.

I thank and acknowledge Dr. JuYoung Park, PhD, Hartford Geriatric Social Work Faculty Scholar, for her devotion and dedication to helping seniors' by finding ways to improve the quality of their lives and for conducting several Florida Atlantic University studies on Sit N Fit Chair Yoga.

And I acknowledge and thank Dr. Ruth McCaffrey, DNP, ARNP, FNP-BC, GNP-BC, for her perseverance, and dedication to conducting studies to obtain scientific evidence proving of the benefits of Sit N Fit Chair Yoga. Thank you also to Bill McCaffrey for sharing his time and expertise in images and document layout.

To all the above I say,

Namaste.

namaste

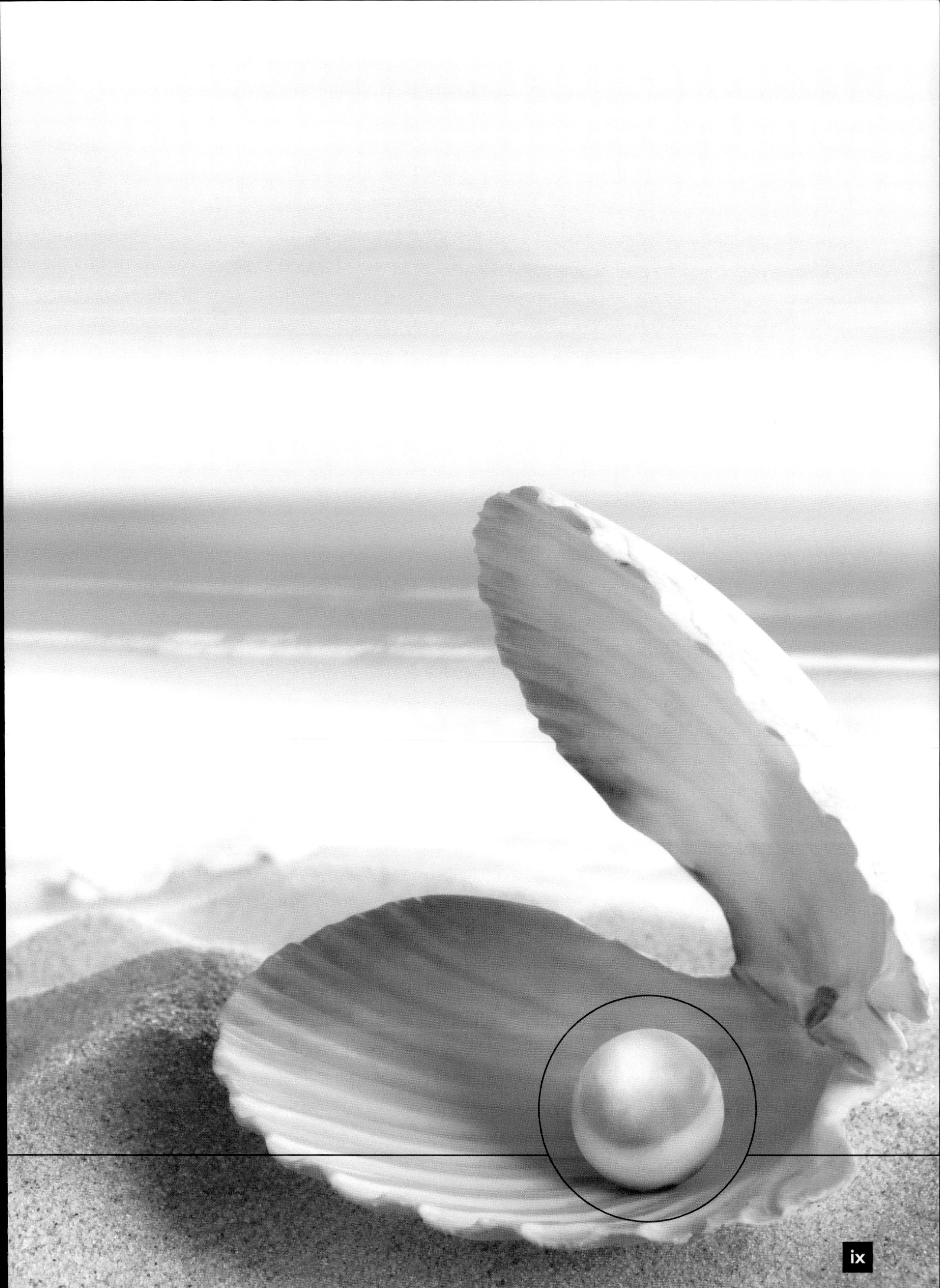

Foreword

Yoga has become a household word across America; yet many still do not know that one does not have to be a flexible contortionist to experience the physical, mental and spiritual benefits of this ancient discipline of conscious living. This book, *Sit N Fit Chair Yoga* by Kristine Lee, is the capstone on her work with students to manage and reduce pain for students challenged with medical conditions that prevents them from doing many of the classic hatha yoga postures. It has been an honor to be one of the yoga instructors in the Florida Atlantic University, Christine E. Lynn College of Nursing research project which has documented evidence of the benefits of the program. The research shows improved physical function and balance as well as increasing well-being. Even the Alzheimer's day center participants showed improved physical function and increased ability to focus their attention and lower anxiety.

To be involved with the Sit N Fit Chair Yoga program is an interesting contrast to my first exposure to yoga in the early 1960's when I looked at the photos in my mother's copy of *The Complete Illustrated Book of Yoga* by Swami Vishnu-devananda. The uniquely attired Indian male model in various odd looking positions intrigued me. At that time yoga was still largely thought of as part of the "counter-culture of the 60's" and there was no chance of finding a yoga instructor in my suburban Midwestern town to investigate my curiosity about yoga; but many years later I received a call from a yoga teacher inviting me to attend her new class at a South Florida wellness center. It was as if peanut found butter when I experienced that first yoga session and I became a dedicated yoga student.

My interest in the amazing power of the holistic science of yoga increased as I reaped the benefits of this transformational and healing way of living. My studies and trainings led to certification as an Integrative Yoga Therapist and a master's degree in psychology focusing on Yoga and Mind/Body Health from Sonoma State University in California. With more than 30 years of personal practice and 25 years of teaching, I have witnessed how yoga has enhanced the well-being of hundreds of people with diverse challenges.

I can confidently recommend this book and the way Kristine organized the structure of this program. The words she chose for the parts of the book are so appropriate for describing what I witnessed in my students during the research project: "The Regenerations," "The Antidotes," "The Revivers," and "The Transformers." The data that has come in through the research confirms what I observed. Many in the program walked through the door the first day struggling with canes and walkers and expressed the fears of moving with their list of aches and pains and apprehensions about doing yoga. To see them gain confidence and be able to do the movements from their secure chairs was amazing. To see the stress fall from their faces was awesome.

Beyond the research data is the joy of observing the calm, centered confidence that grew during the two month, twice weekly program. The eldest member of the group, an 84-year-old retired attorney, told me the breathing exercises have made a significant difference in his life. The smile on his face as he expressed that to me was priceless.

Finding a tool to ease the stress in life is important at any age, but so valuable when one is faced with issues of aging often combined with various aches and pains and challenges of standing and walking. Many of the students improved enough to do some of the standing poses with the chair beside them.

Even if you are a seasoned yogi without physical limitations this is a good read. It is a great practice for those captive to a chair in an office, sitting at an airport terminal, sitting on a plane, and a host of other creative places. It is perfect for caregivers — both the givers and the cared for.

One of my favorite quotes about yoga is from T. K.V. Desikachar's book *The Heart of Yoga: Developing a Personal Practice*; I find it particularly relevant to students beginning the practice of hatha yoga later in life with challenges that might keep them from attempting even a chair yoga class. He says: "We begin where we are and how we are, and whatever happens, happens." I recommend reading *Sit N Fit Chair Yoga* and giving the practice a try; I think you will love what happens.

Diane Zantop, MA
Integrative Yoga Therapist
Boca Raton, Florida

Introduction: THE REGENERATIONS

The Sit N Fit Chair Yoga program was created to manage and reduce pain due to medical conditions such as osteoarthritis and to give those who could not do standing exercise the full experience of a yoga class while sitting in a chair. **Some of the benefits include:**

- *Increasing oxygenation*
- *Eliciting the relaxation response*
- *Correcting posture*
- *Increasing circulation, flexibility, balance and strength*

The movements are progressive, comprehensive, and sequenced for greatest ease and benefit. The practice was developed to open and create space where the natural pull of gravity has compressed or constricted space. This allows oxygen and blood to go into the cells and nourish them. The lymphatic system is also stimulated, detoxifying and cleansing the cells. By increasing circulation, all the systems, glands, hormones, and organs of the body are able to function more efficiently. Sit N Fit Chair Yoga elicits the relaxation response releasing stress, tension, and emotional trauma that can be held in our cells from going through our everyday life.

The yoga practice is personalized. Every student is instructed to "listen to your body" and "work your edge, the point of gentle resistance." However, if you feel pain, you should stop, relax, and breathe. Students may modify the pose to accommodate their body, or simply visualize the pose. It is not necessary to do every pose in every class. It is recommended that the spine be taken in every direction in every class. As students progress, and only if it is appropriate, the standing poses can replace the identical seated poses. For safety, use a sturdy non-collapsible chair.

Soothing music played during the class calms anxiety, helps students focus, and enables suggestions and visualizations to be recorded in the students' subconscious mind. The result is pain reduction, enhanced strength and mobility, and improved quality of life.

Florida Atlantic University conducted two research studies on Sit N Fit Chair Yoga. Focus group data analysis on the 2011 Sit N Fit Chair Yoga pilot study showed pain reduction, improved mobility, a feeling of security and improvement in sense of well-being. Group comments included: "It makes my body feel better and I have less pain." "I feel better in terms of my ability to do more things at home." "I learned how to relax, which I didn't really know how before. I learned how it makes your body feel better." "Nothing in my situation has changed but my attitude toward my life has changed for the better. I am more calm."[1]

Additional research at FAU continued on Sit N Fit Chair Yoga with a larger group in 2012. The study results showed significant improvement in depression and life satisfaction.[2] Data analyzed on older adults with moderate and severe Alzheimer's Disease showed significant improvement in balance, gait speed, walking ability as well as increased focus and concentration.[3]

In 2013 Florida Atlantic University received funding for a two-year study (2014-2015): "The Effect of Sit N Fit Chair Yoga Among Community Dwelling Older Adults with Osteoarthritis" supported by the National Center for Complementary and Alternative Medicine of the National Institutes of Health. The study is ongoing at the time of publication of this book and will measure both physiologic and psychosocial outcomes associated with the Sit N Fit Chair Yoga program. Physical measures include pain, balance, gait speed and walking ability. Psychosocial measures include emotional distress and depression, life satisfaction, fatigue and the ability to participate in social interactions.

Part 1: THE REVIVERS

BREATH OF LIFE 5 to10 minutes (one breathing technique per class)

3-Part Yogic Breathing

Americans generally use 10% of their lungs. Diaphragmatic breathing retrains students to:

- *Use the full capacity of the lungs*
- *Strengthen the lungs*
- *Elicit the relaxation response*
- *Calm the mind*

1. Sit tall with a straight spine. When you fill up your lungs with air, they take up more space; the diaphragm is pushed down and this makes the belly rise. Allow this motion to happen. Place your fingertips gently on your belly and relax your abdominal muscles. In yoga we breathe through the nostrils unless instructed otherwise. This helps slow down and purify the breath as it passes through the nostril hairs. Take a deep breath in through both nostrils. As you do this, allow the belly to rise into the hands. Take a long slow exhalation. Gently press all the stale air out of the lungs, never forcing or straining, "steady and comfortable" is the mantra. Repeat this for three breaths.

2. Now gently place your fingertips on your ribcage. Take a deep breath. Allow the belly to rise and the ribcage to open. Slowly exhale. Gently press all the stale air out of the lungs on the exhale. Repeat this three times and make your exhalation a little longer than your inhalation.

3. Gently place your fingertips on your upper chest. Take a deep breath. Allow the belly to rise, the ribcage to open, and the upper chest to lift. As you exhale allow the chest to fall, the ribcage to close, and the belly to recede. Repeat this three times. Make your exhalation a little longer than your inhalation. Once you have mastered this, you can start with #3, relaxing your hands on your belly or resting the back of your hands on your thighs.

This breathing technique is also a great breath to do while lying down. If your mind will not quiet at bedtime, use this breath to help you get to sleep. Remember to slow down the breath, and when the mind begins to wonder to thoughts, bring your attention back to the breath. You may want to visualize a healing white light coming into your cells on the inhalation, and a gray mist leaving you on the exhalation. This breathing exercise will help you let go of negativity.

Alternate Nostril Breathing

Benefits include:

- *Enhances concentration*
- *Quiets the mind, aka "the committee in the head"*
- *Balances the right and left sides of the brain*
- *Helps gain mental clarity*

Alternate nostril breathing balances the right and left sides of the brain. In Chinese medicine this is referred to as the Yin Yang principle and in healthy organisms these two forces are balanced. Yoga balances the mind and the body, and the breath is the thread that connects the mind to the body.

Sit with a straight spine. Raise your right hand and turn your palm toward your face. Bend your index finger and your middle finger and place the tip of these fingers into your palm. Use your ring finger and your thumb to close off your nostrils. If you have difficulty using the ring finger and thumb, keep all fingers straight and use the outside of your index finger and your thumb.

Imagine that you have a candle in front of you and that your breath is so light it does not flicker the flame. You will be slowing down the breath. When you slow down the breath, you slow down the mind. This quiets the "committee in the head" and enhances concentration.

1. Take a deep breath in through both nostrils.
2. Close your right nostril off with your thumb and breathe out through your left nostril.
3. Breathe in through your left nostril, close your left nostril with your ring finger.
4. Release your thumb and exhale through your right nostril.
5. Inhale through your right nostril, close your right nostril with your thumb, release your ring finger and exhale through your left nostril.

Continue alternating the breath for three to five minutes. Once mastered, this breath can be done for any length of time and is often used as a precursor to meditation.

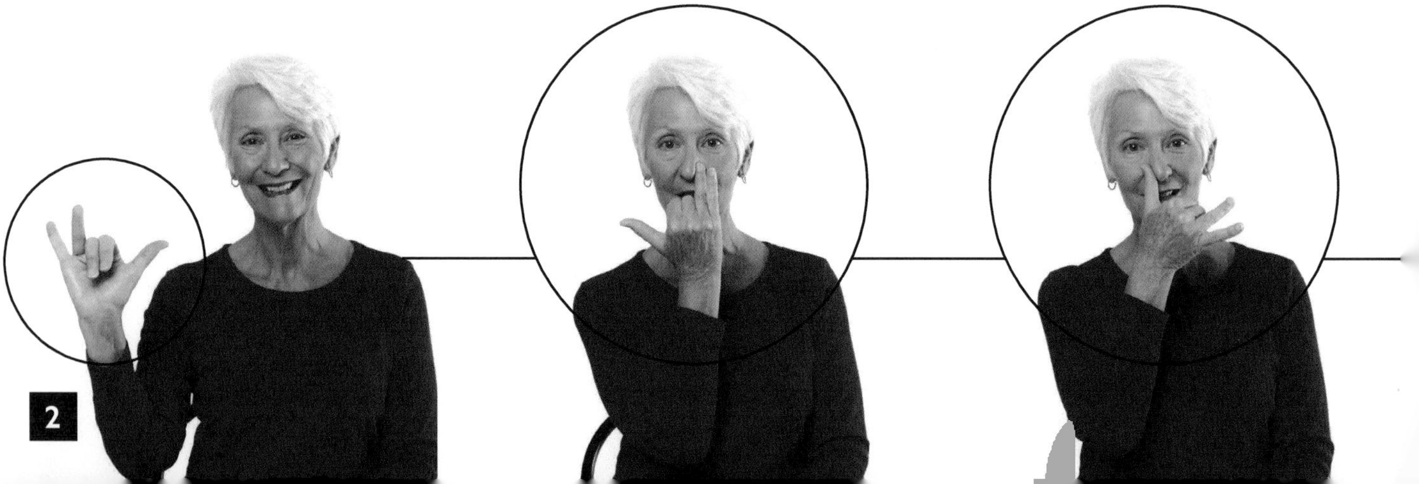

Ujjayi Breath

Benefits include:

- ***Lengthens the breath***
- ***Strengthens and purifies the lungs by expelling carbon dioxide***
- ***Teaches breath control***
- ***Produces heat in the body for enhanced flexibility***
- ***Tones the abdominal muscles***

Begin with a straight spine. It is easiest to learn this technique with the mouth open. Once mastered, you may close the mouth.

1. To begin, take a deep breath in through your nostrils. Open your mouth and whisper the sound of "Ah" as you exhale, gently pressing all the stale air out of your lungs. Your navel will gently press toward your spine. Never force or strain; the mantra is "steady and comfortable."

2. As you inhale, whisper the sound of "Ah," and imagine that you are sucking through a straw. That is the motion in the throat. The back of the tongue lifts slightly and there is a slight constriction in the back of the throat and in the abdominal region.

3. Exhale whispering the sound "Ah."

Repeat steps 2 and 3 and continue for three to five minutes.

This technique teaches breath control. When you control your breath, you control your mind and become more focused and calm.

steady and comfortable

Part 2: THE ANTIDOTES

THE BODY PROPER Seated Poses – 20 to 25 minutes

Seated Mountain

Corrects posture and enhances ability to breathe

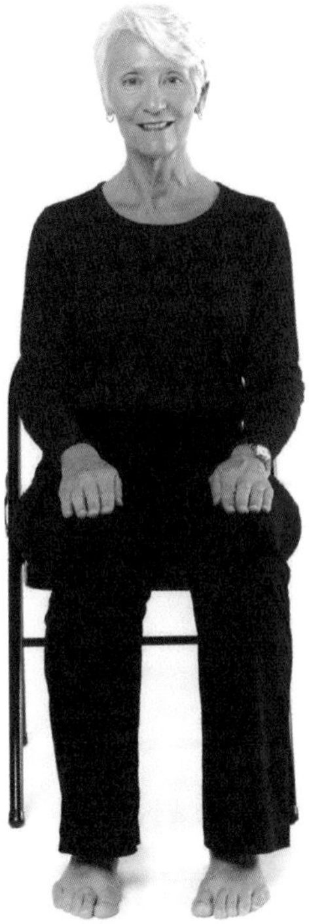

Begin with a straight spine and correct posture. Toes in front of heels, knees in line with hips, lift ribcage, sternum, lift shoulders up, back, then down, and lift crown (top center) of head.

Relax shoulders down away from ears.

JOINT ROTATIONS

Shoulder Rolls

Relieves joint pain and increases circulation

Circle shoulders forward, up, back and down, then reverse, rotating shoulders. Place fingers on shoulders and circle elbows forward, up, back and down, then reverse.

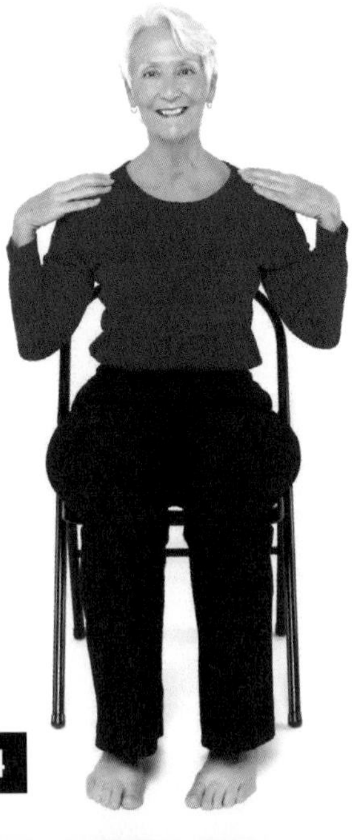

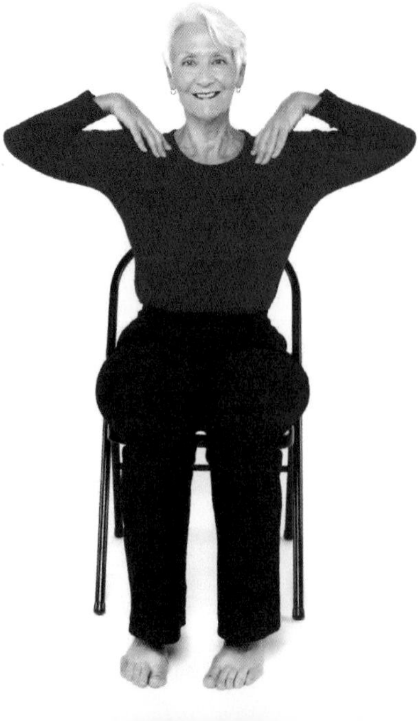

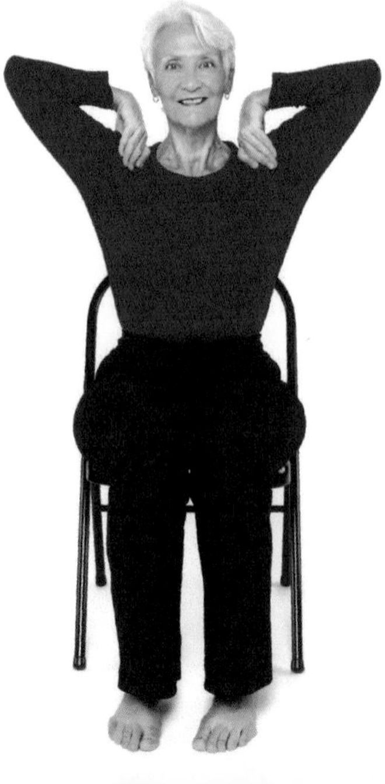

Foot Circles

Lift right foot and circle 3 times clockwise then counter clockwise rotating ankles.
Repeat with left foot.

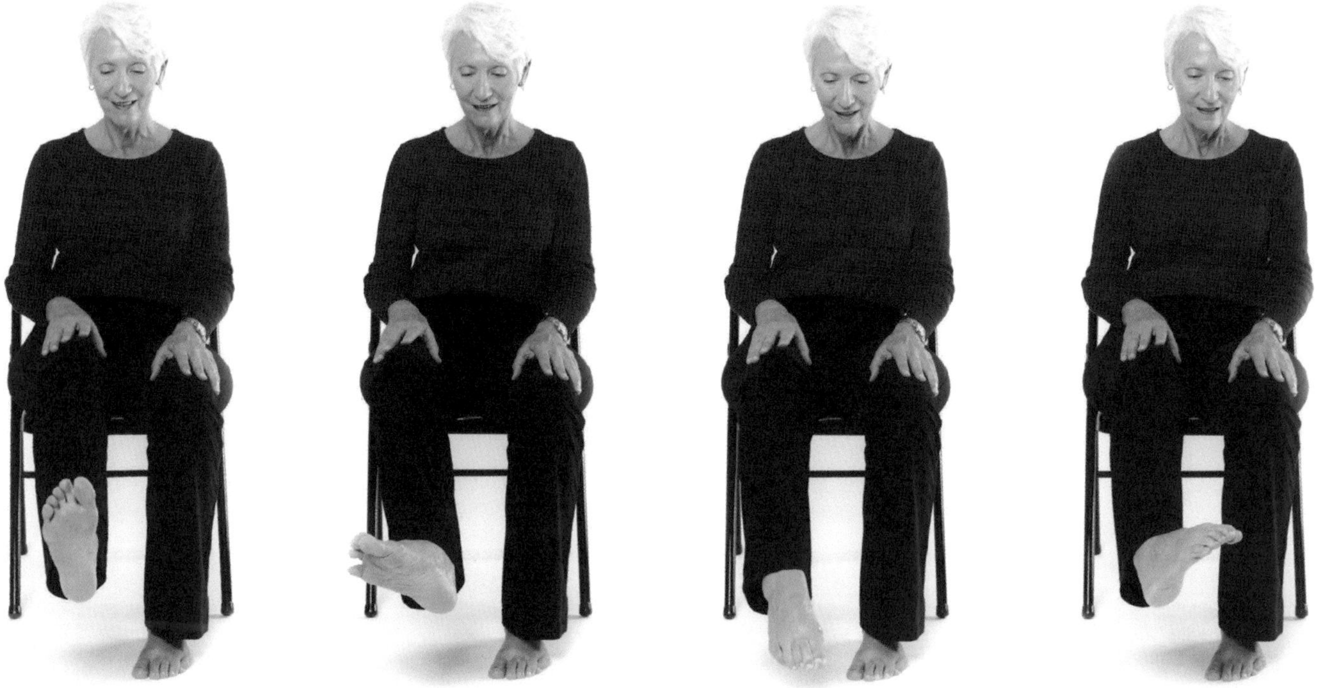

Hip Rotation

Hold right knee with right hand, lift foot up (or foot can remain on the floor if necessary) and slowly make a circle with the knee, 3 times clockwise then counter clockwise, repeat with left knee.

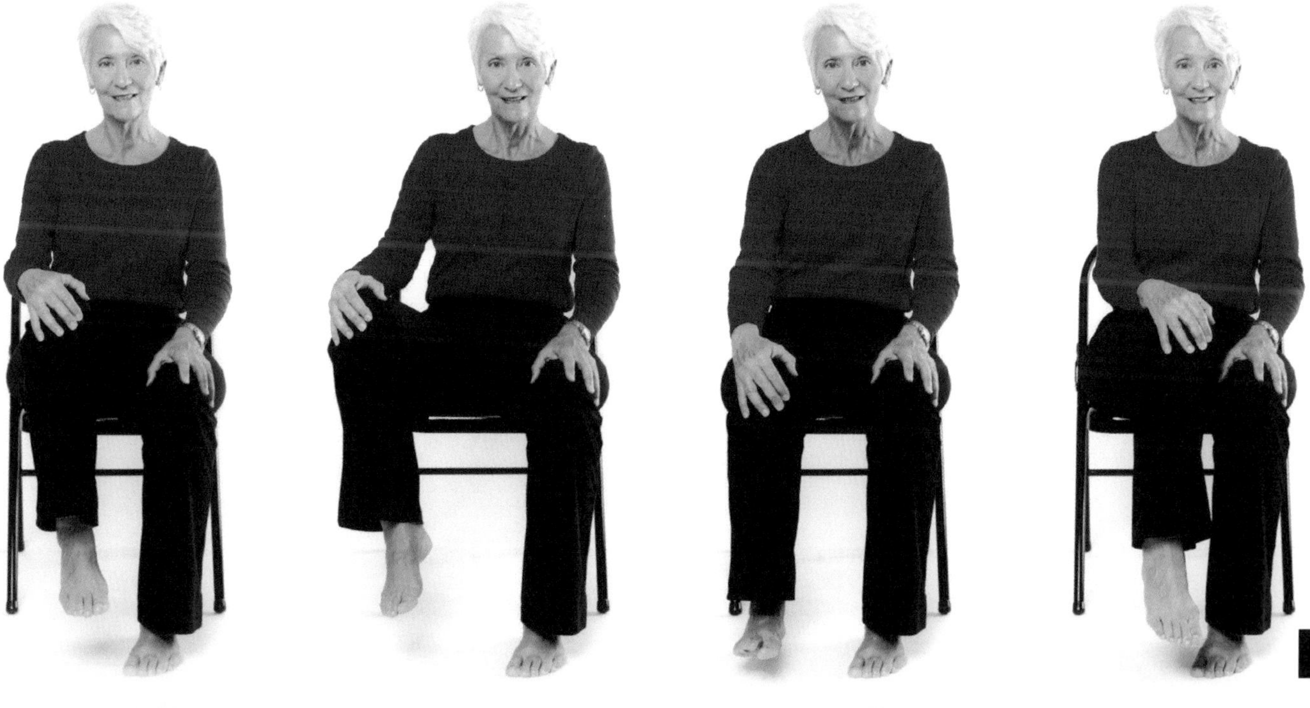

Fist Circles

Rotating wrists both directions. Circle to the right 3 times, then reverse.

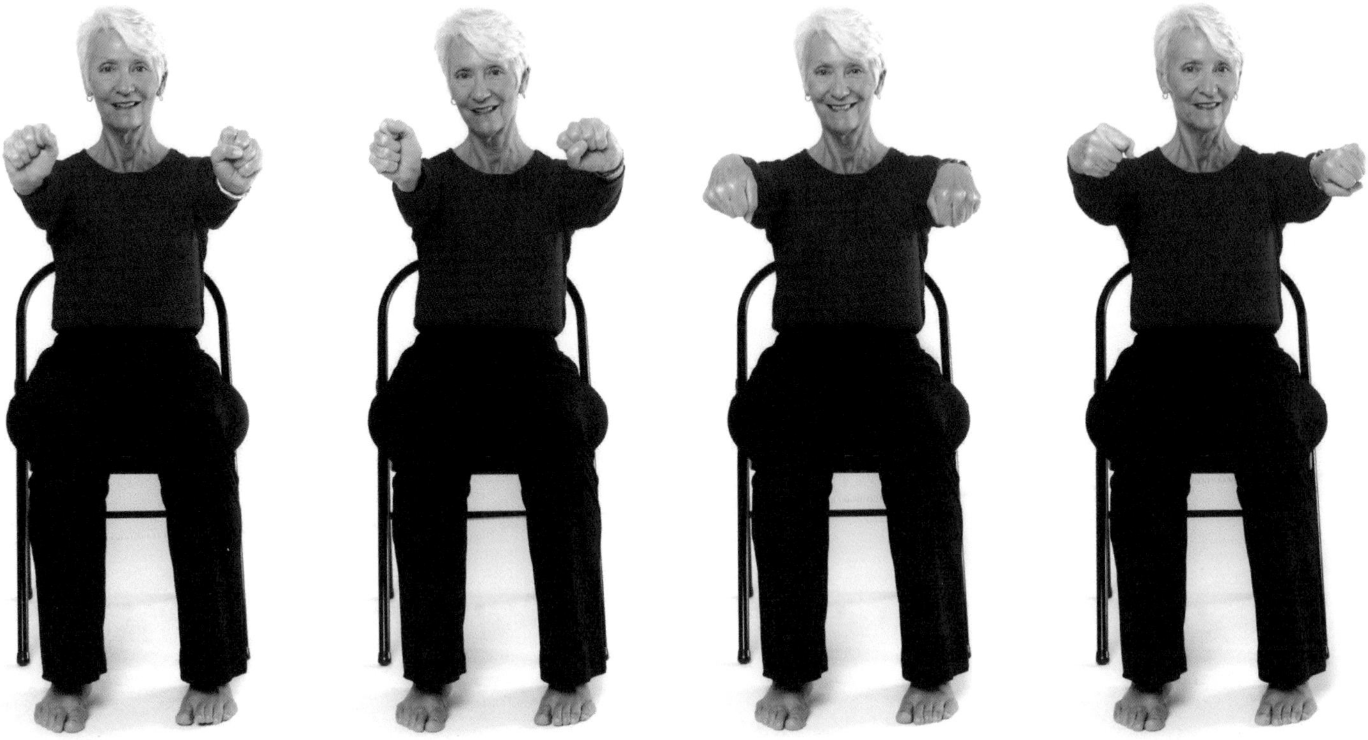

Arm and Shoulder Toner

Press heels of the hands forward straight out from your shoulders, then move the fingers to the right, back up, then to the left. Repeat 3 times.

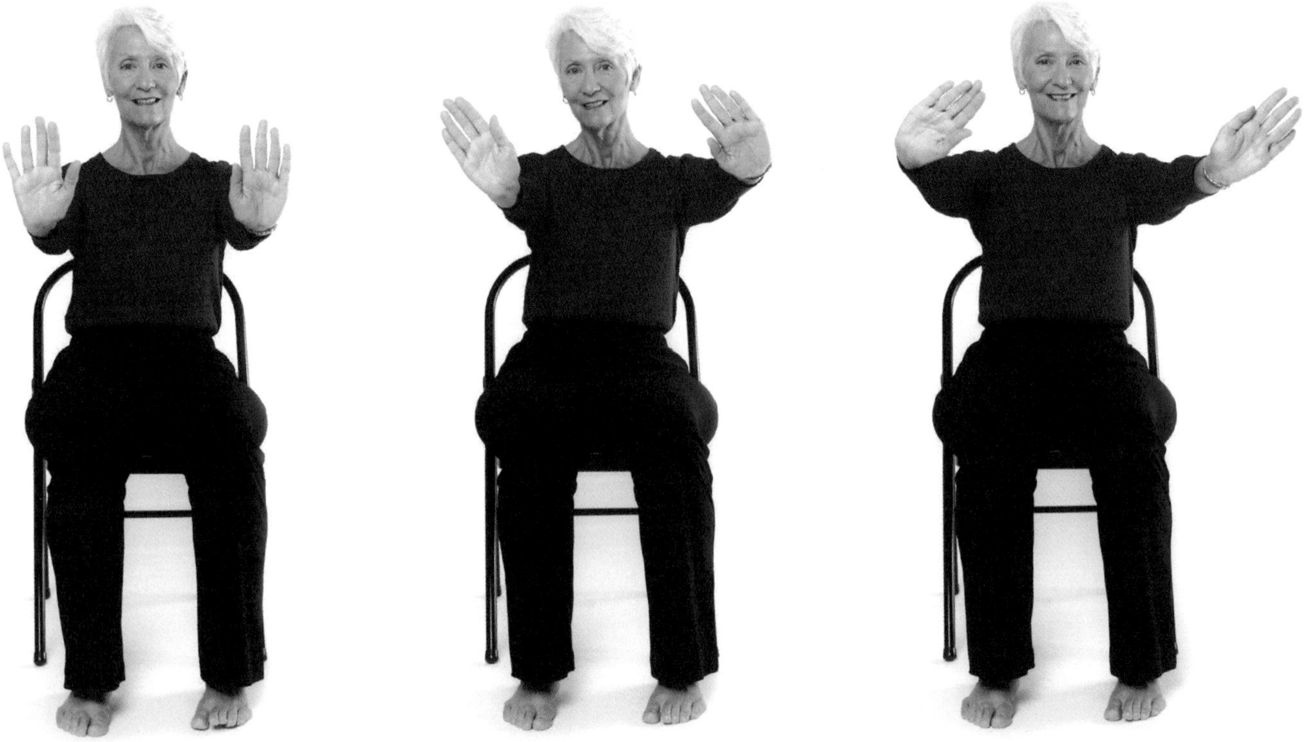

Eye Revivers

Exercises the optic muscles and relieves fatigued eyes

With your eyes, trace the face of a clock slowly, reverse direction. Look up, to the sides and down as far as possible.

Trace the face of a clock with your eyes. Look 12, 3, 6, 9 o'clock then back up to 12 o'clock. Then reverse direction.

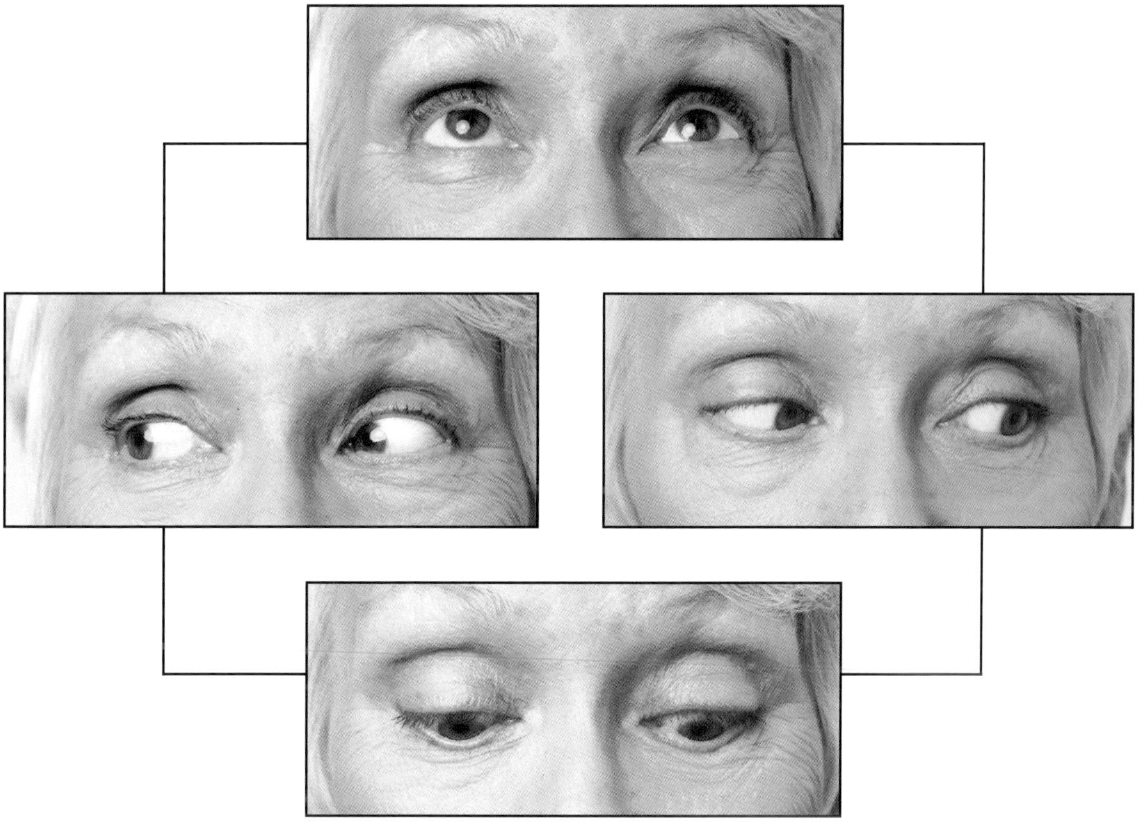

Zig-zag the eyes – Upper right, lower left – 3 times, then upper left, lower right, 3 times.

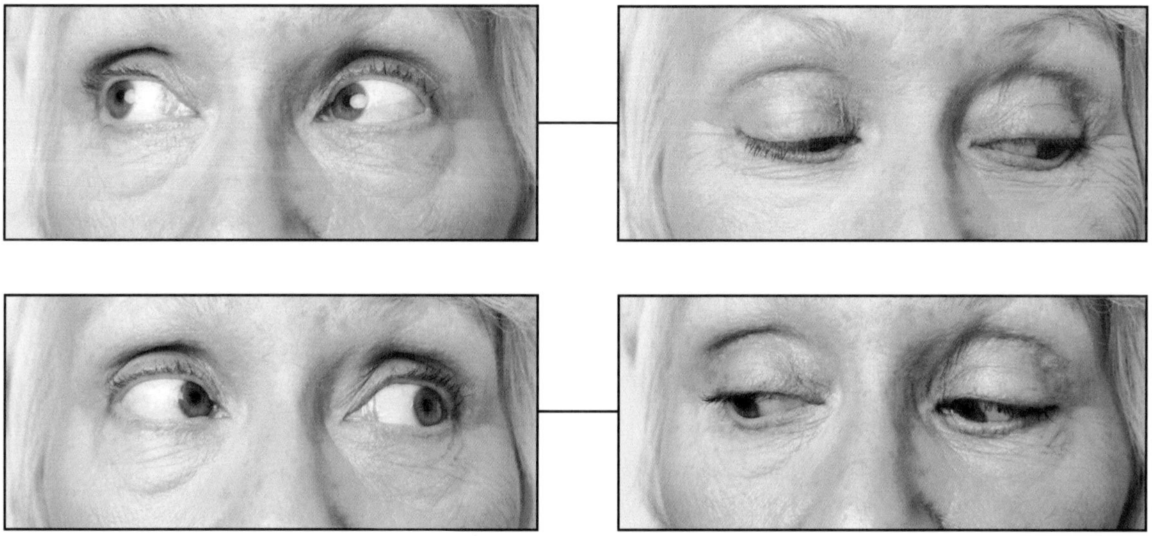

Spinal Lubricator

Start with a straight tall spine, hands on hips. Lean forward to the right, lean forward center, lean forward left, lean back, taking the torso in a circle. Reverse the direction and repeat.

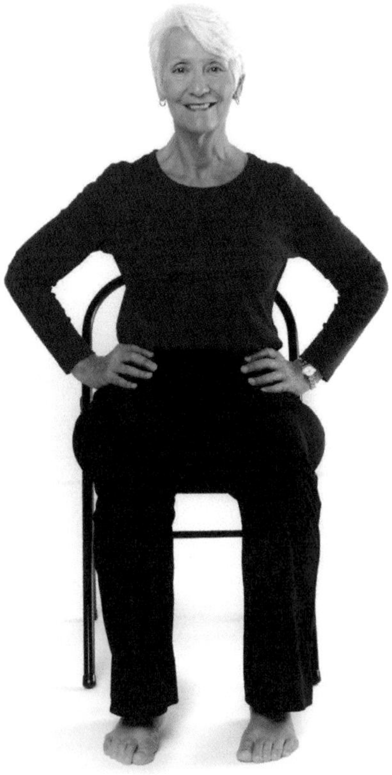

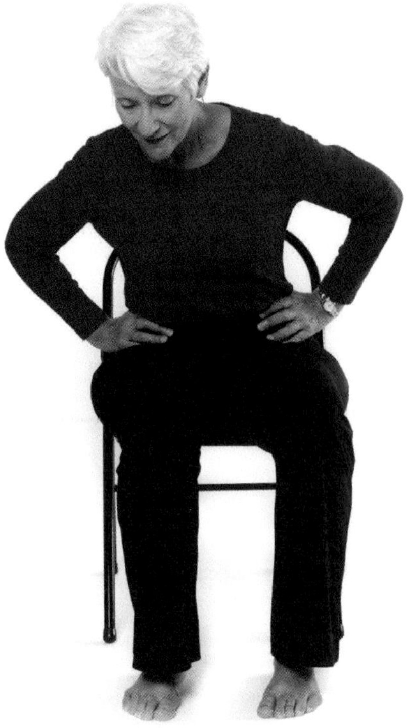

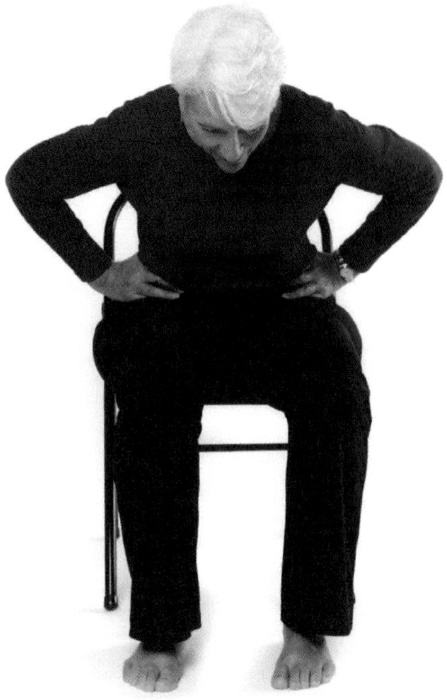

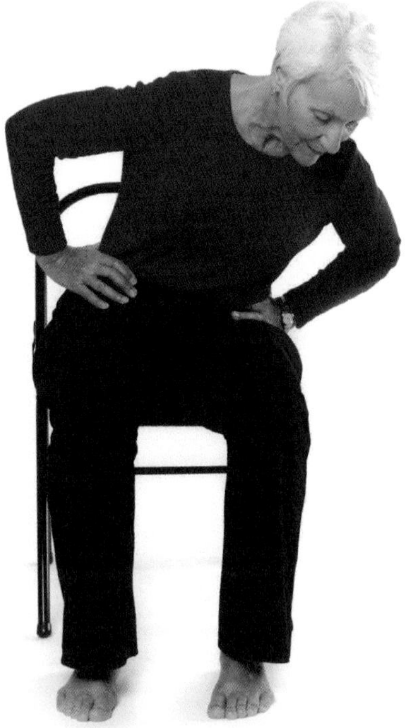

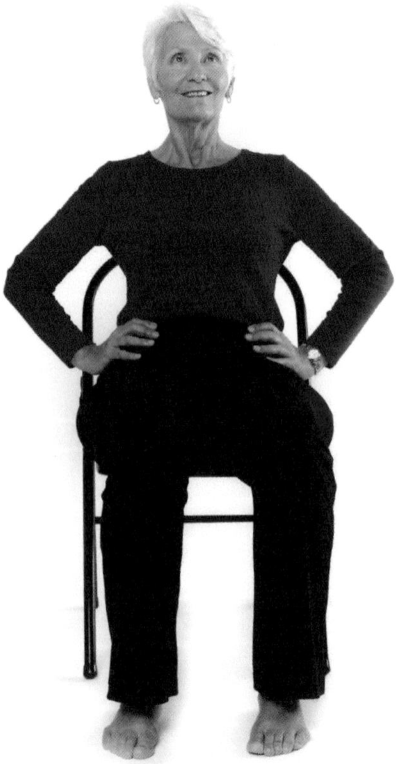

Spinal Twist

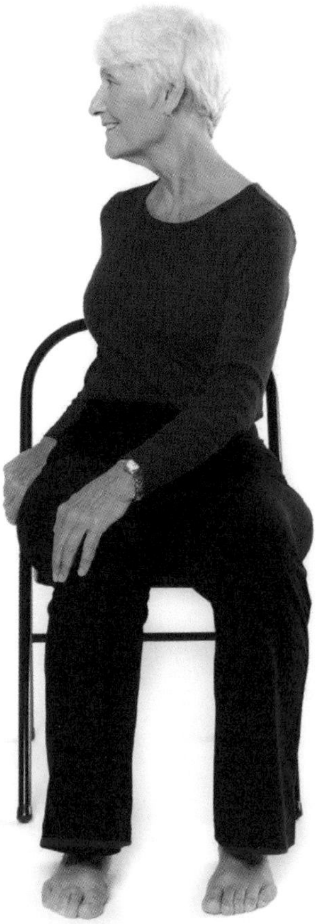

Benefits include:

- *Tones abdominal muscles*
- *Increases spinal health and flexibility*
- *Massages internal organs and stimulates digestion*
- *Increases space and right alignment of spine*
- *Releases stress and tension*

Start with legs in line with hips and sit tall. Take right hand and hold the right side or back of the chair. Turn the torso towards the right slowly and allow hips to rotate slightly with spine. Take left hand outside right knee or thigh. The rotation comes from the hips, then the ribcage, then the chest. Let the head naturally follow the spine.

Coming out of the twist, release both hands and arms, move the chest, ribcage then hips left, back to the center. Repeat to the left.

For variations, cross ankles or knees and repeat both directions.

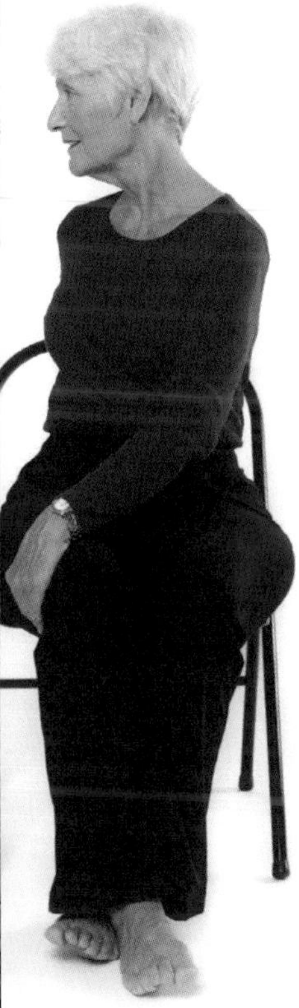

Spinal Twist ankles crossed
Cross right ankle over left, twist to the right.
Left ankle over right, twist to the left.

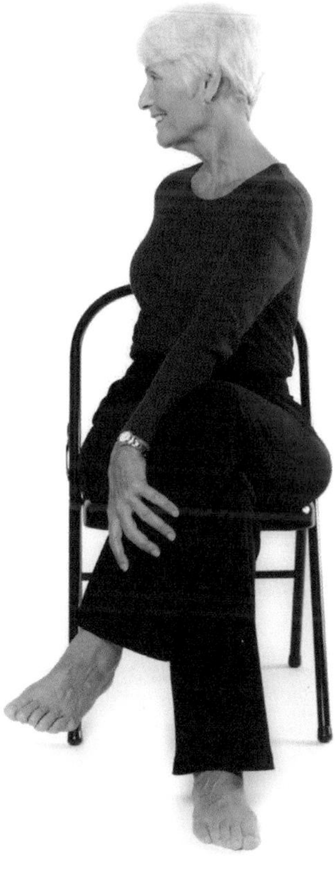

Spinal Twist knees crossed open belly
Crossing the left leg over right when twisting to the right, will protect the low spine from over compressing. Reverse.

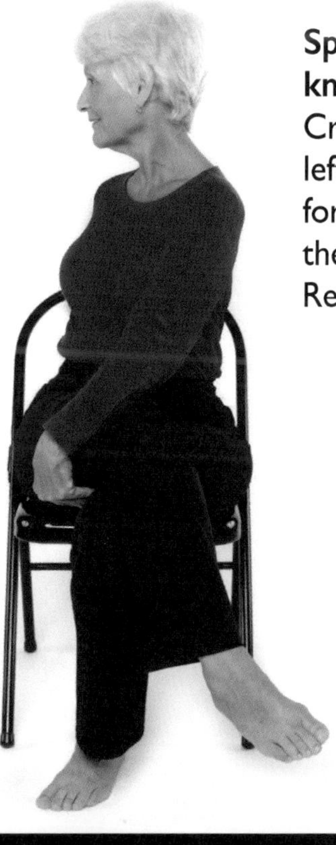

Spinal Twist knees crossed
Cross right leg over left when turning right for a deeper twist in the entire spine. Reverse.

Cervical Vertebra Release

Benefits include:

- *Releases stress*
- *Lengthens the muscles that connect the head to the neck and shoulders*
- *Creates space between the vertebrae*

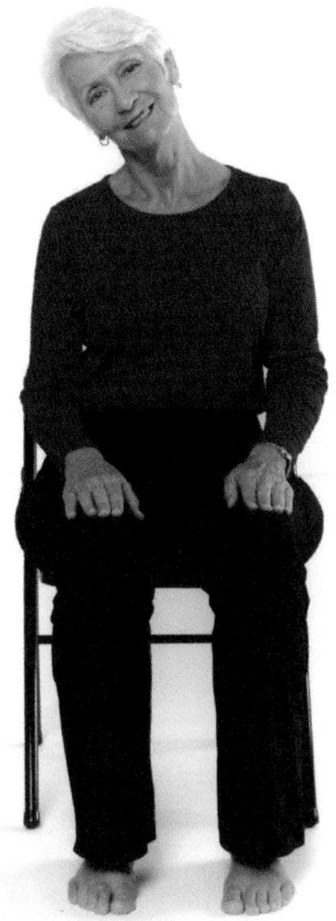

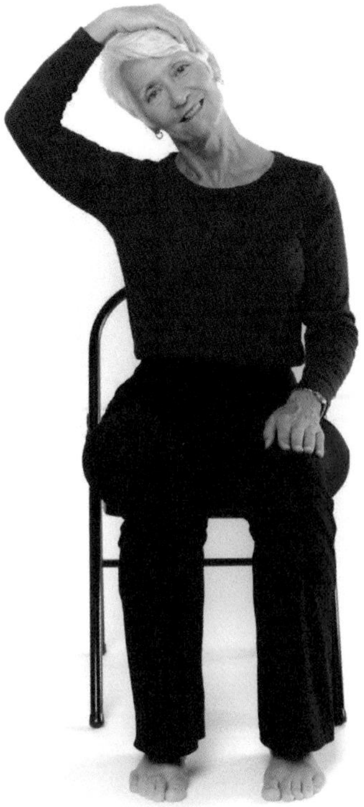

Bring right ear towards right shoulder, lower left shoulder, inhale right hand up, place on left temple, let the weight of the hand and gravity increase the stretch in the left shoulder and neck. Reverse.

Finger Flicks

Hands forward straight out from shoulders, flick fingers out from thumbs several times.

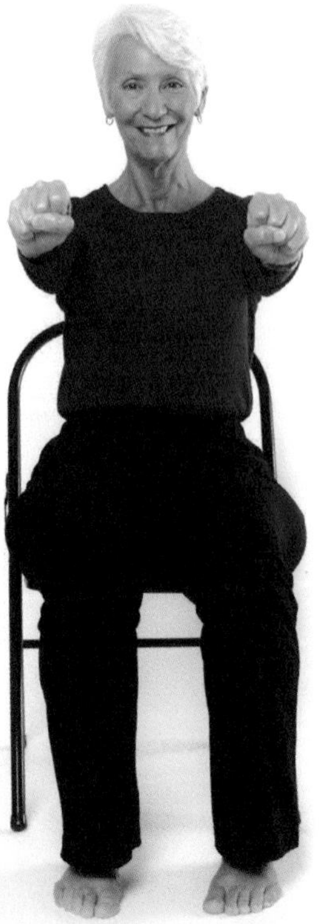

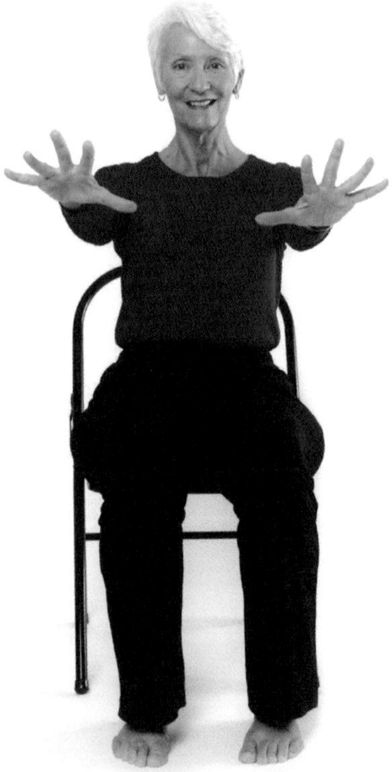

Hand Wake-up

Imagine you have water on your fingers, shake hands to release the water.
Shake fingers up and down.

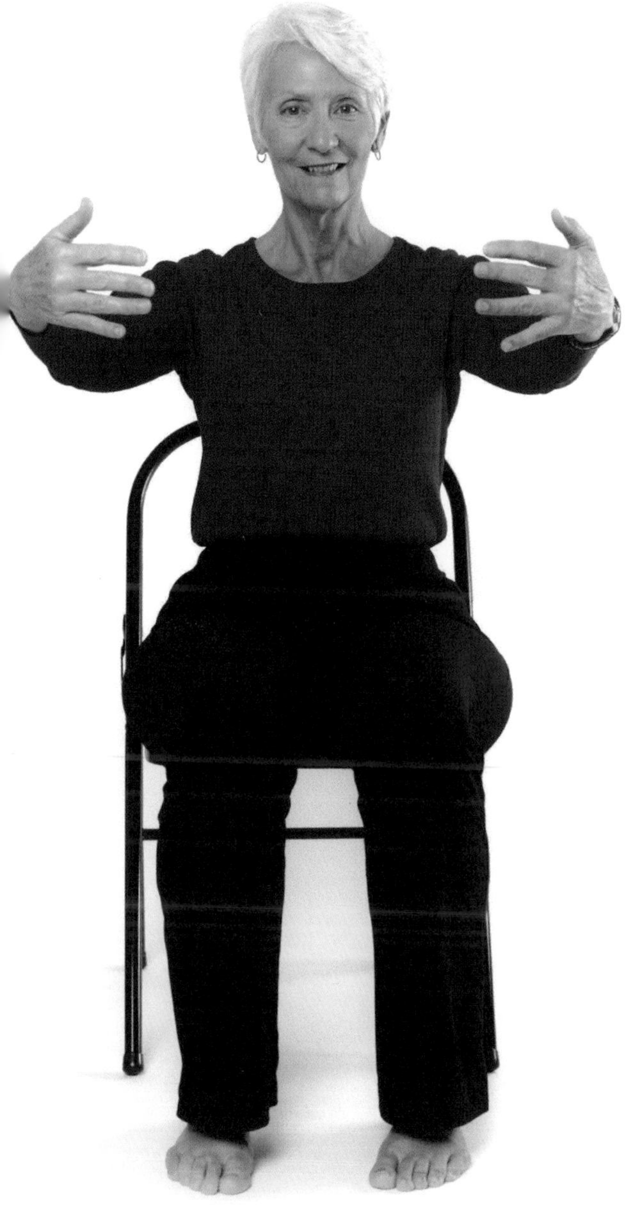

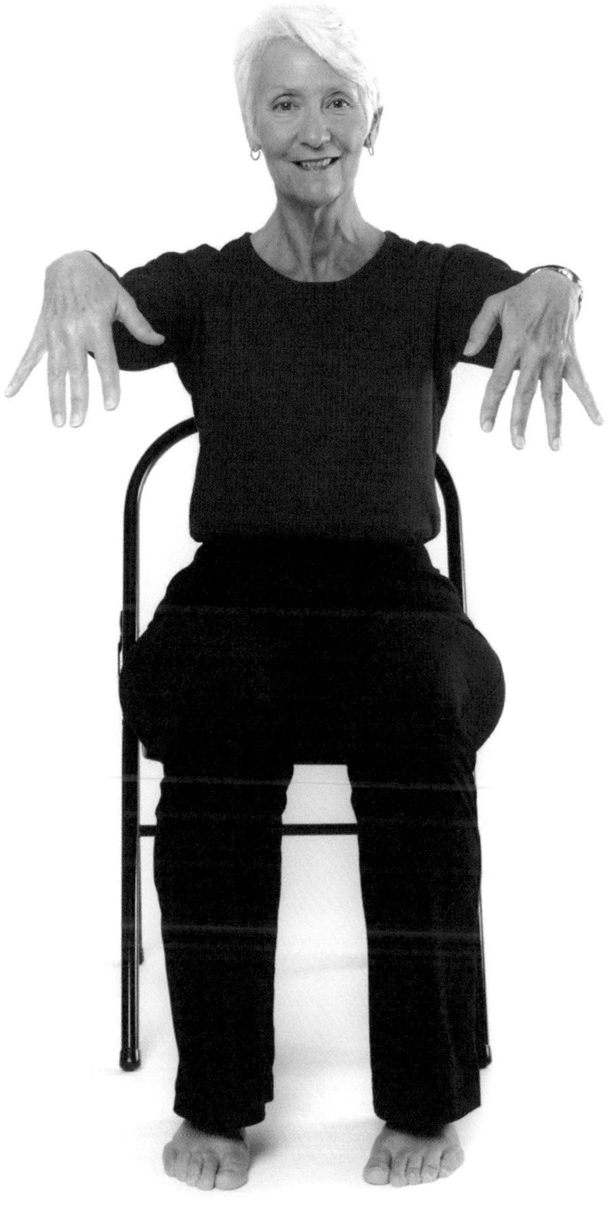

extend and release

Eagle

Benefits include:

- ***Opens shoulders and stretches back muscles located by the shoulder blades***
- ***Opens hips if legs are crossed***

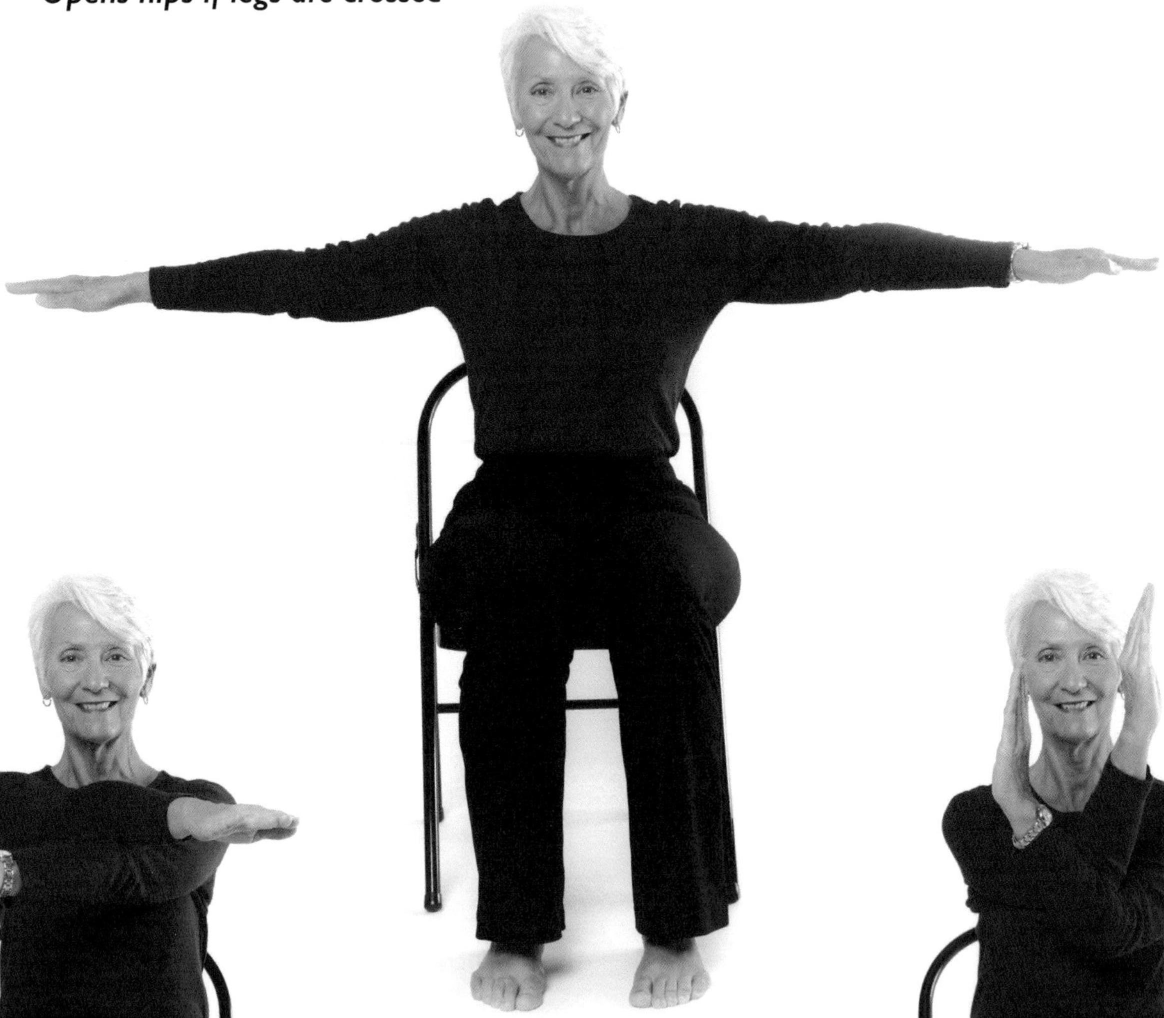

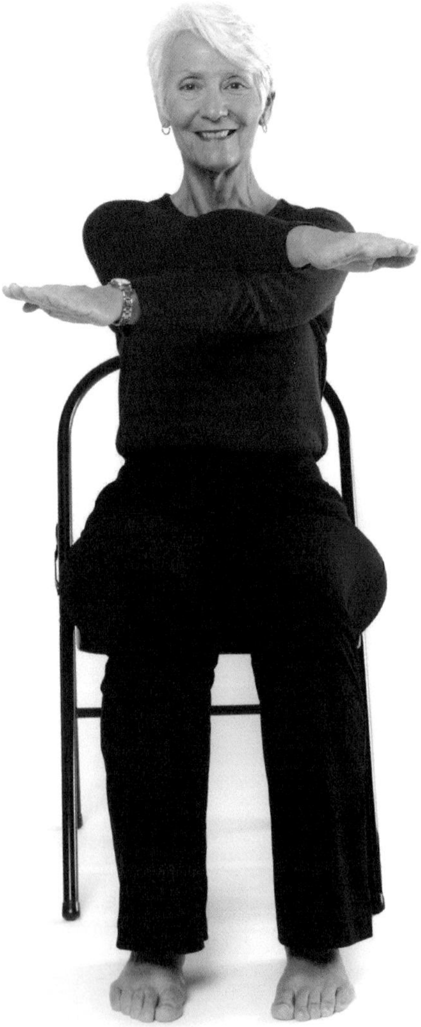

Bring arms straight out from shoulders in a T position.

Keep legs in line with hips or cross ankles or legs for more challenge.

Cross right arm on top of left arm, cross arms at elbows or forearms, lift forearms and hands up, bring backs of hands towards each other, or to touch, or palms together.

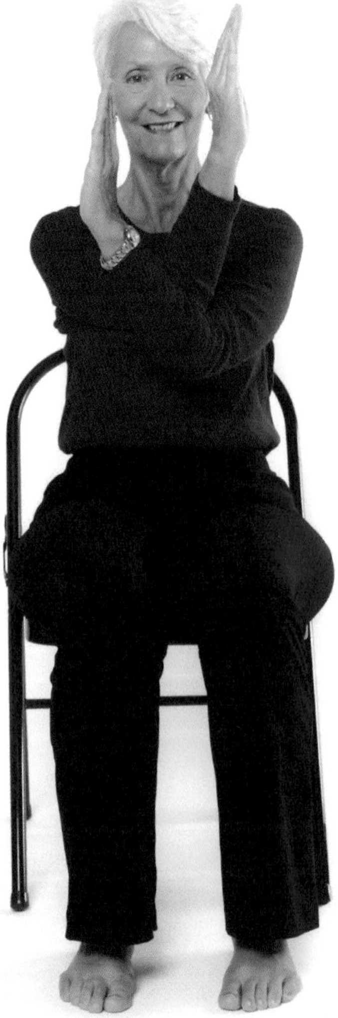

Lift hands up and down slowly. Circle elbows slowly each direction. Bring arms down towards legs. Tuck tailbone, navel up (tilt pelvis) slowly come up. Release arms.

Reverse: left arm on top of right arm, cross arms at elbows or forearms, lift forearms and hands up, bring backs of hands towards each other, or to touch, or palms together.

You may also cross the legs to open the hips. When left arm is on top, cross right leg over left. When right arm is on top, cross left leg over right.

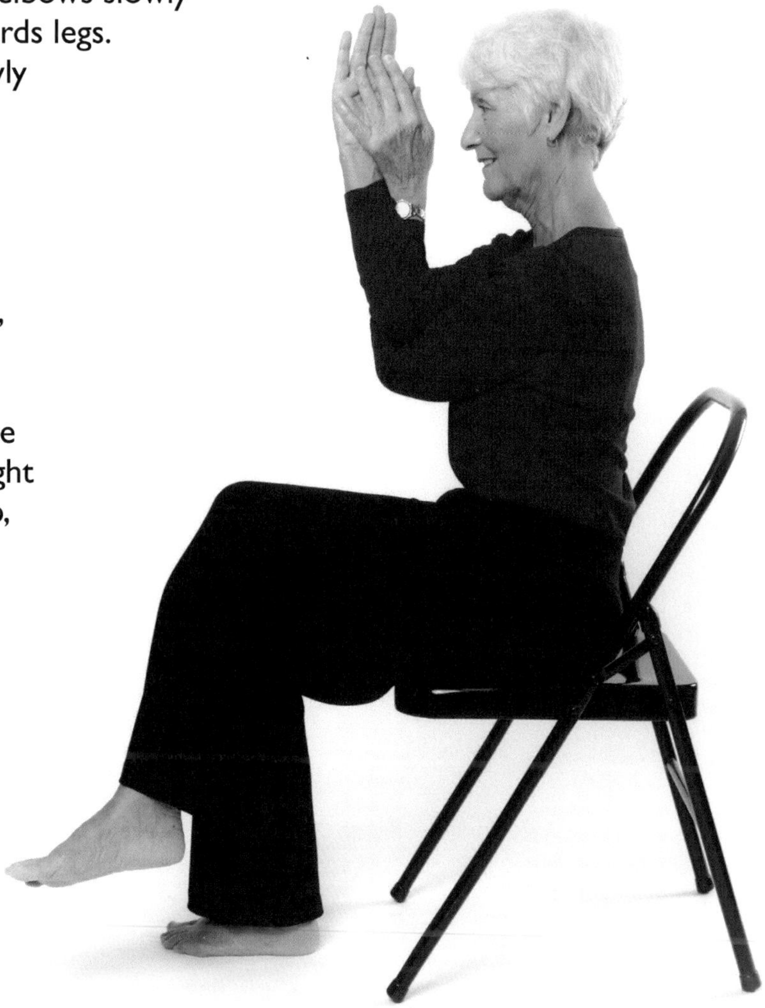

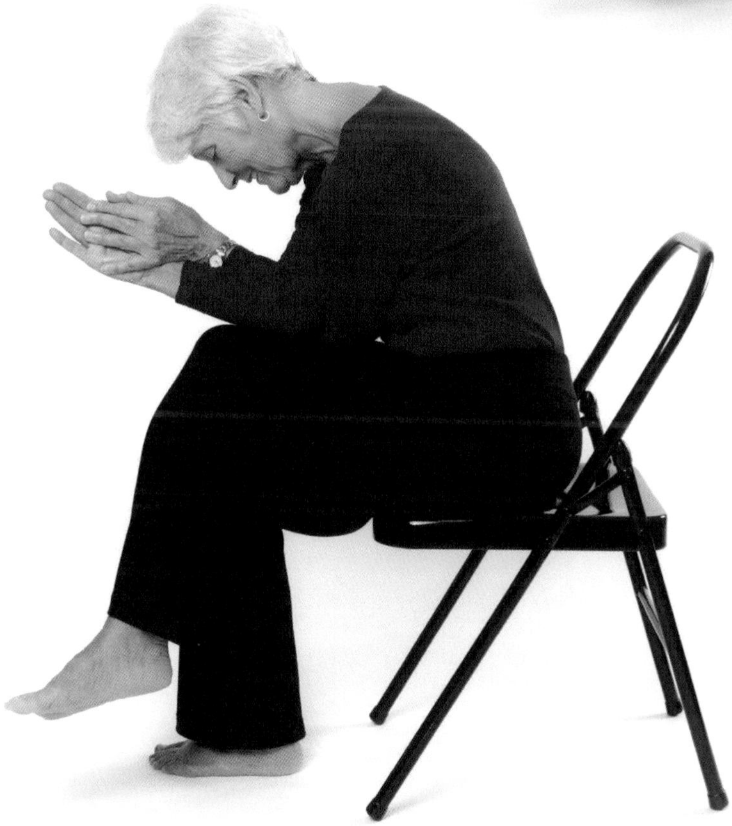

Sun Breath

Benefits include:

- *Stretches arms and shoulders*
- *Relaxes the body*

Palms together over heart, inhale hands and arms up over head, open hands and arms out in a T position, turn palms down, and return palms together over heart. Do two times.

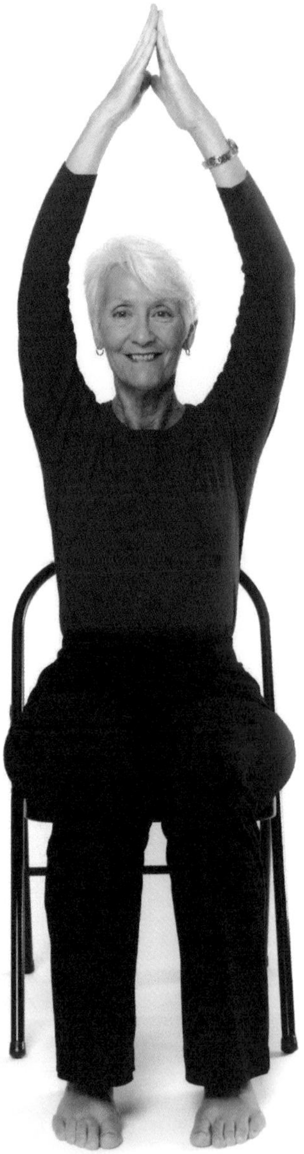

Reverse. Inhale hands together over heart, bring hands down towards lap, open hands, turn palms up and arms out in a T position, palms facing up. Bring hands and arms over head, bring palms together and exhale hands and arms down, returning palms together over heart. Repeat.

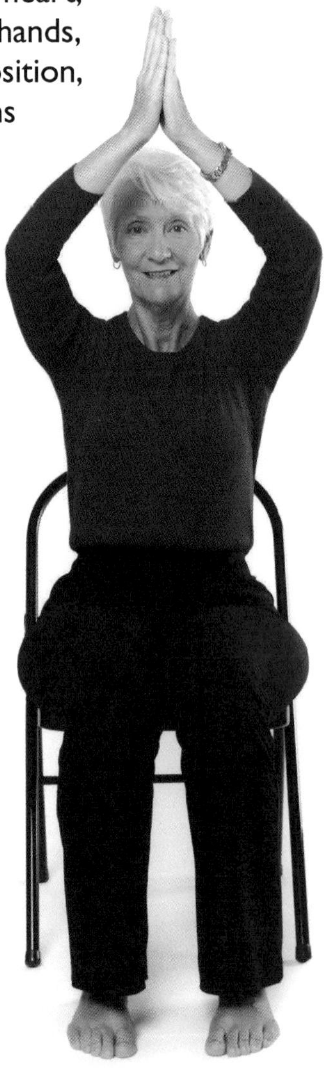

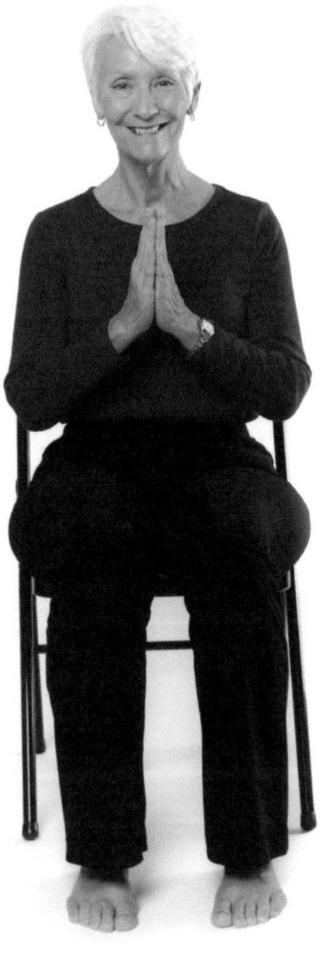

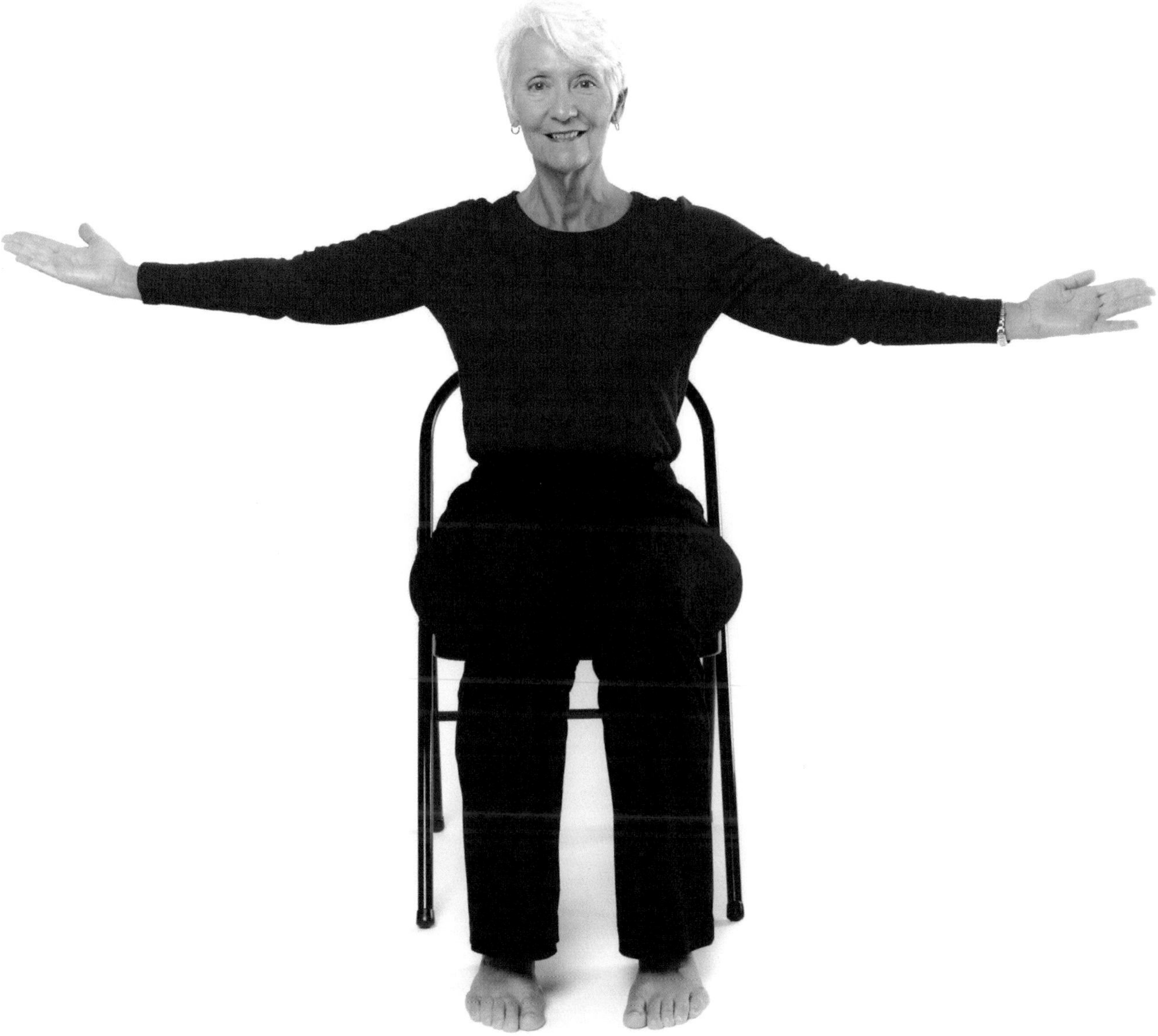

stretch and relax

Stick

Strengthens quadriceps

Lift right leg, flex foot and press through heel, tighten muscles. Hold and breathe.

Repeat with left leg.

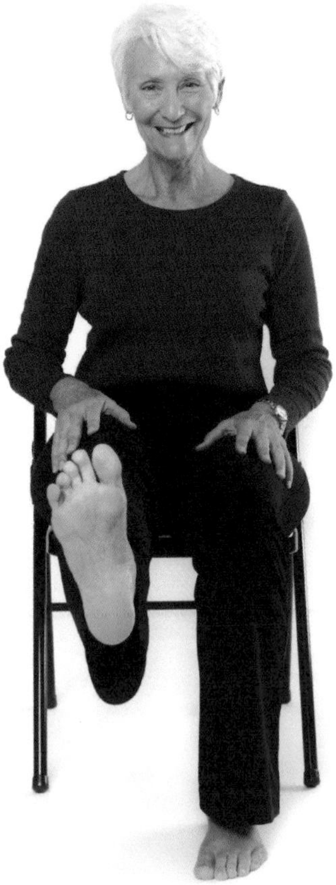

Shin and Calf Toner

Tones shins and calves

Lift toes, heels down. Reverse, lift heels toes down, squeeze calves, repeat several times.

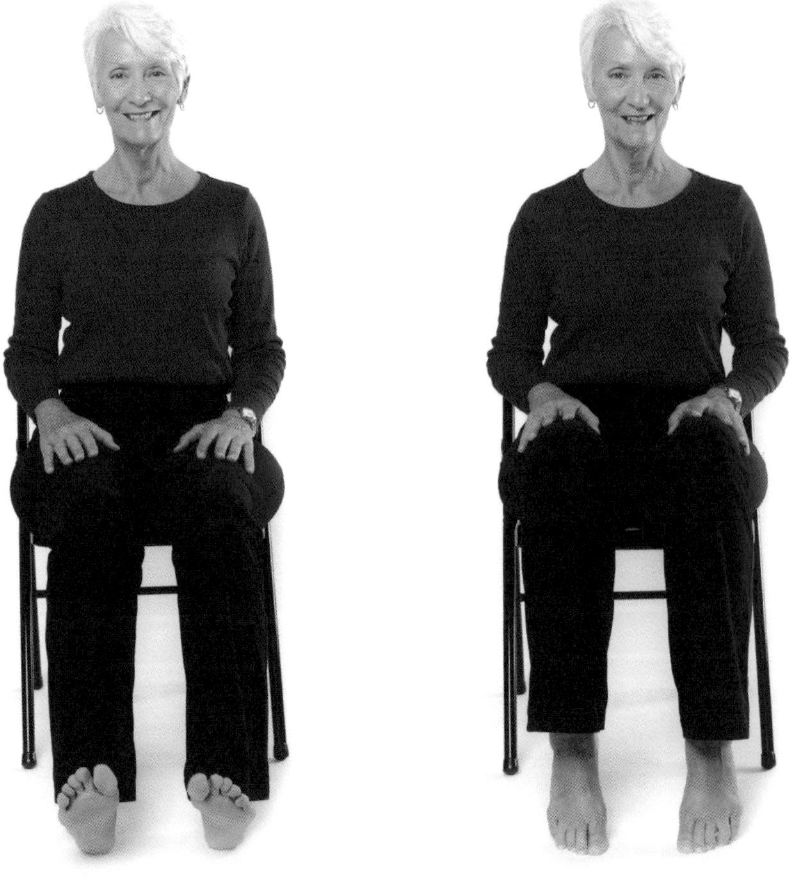

Head to Knee

Stretches back muscles

Lift right knee, bring head toward knee, relax shoulders down, chin towards chest.

Lower leg, press navel in towards spine, and with chin tucked towards chest, slowly come up, lift head up last.

Repeat with left leg.

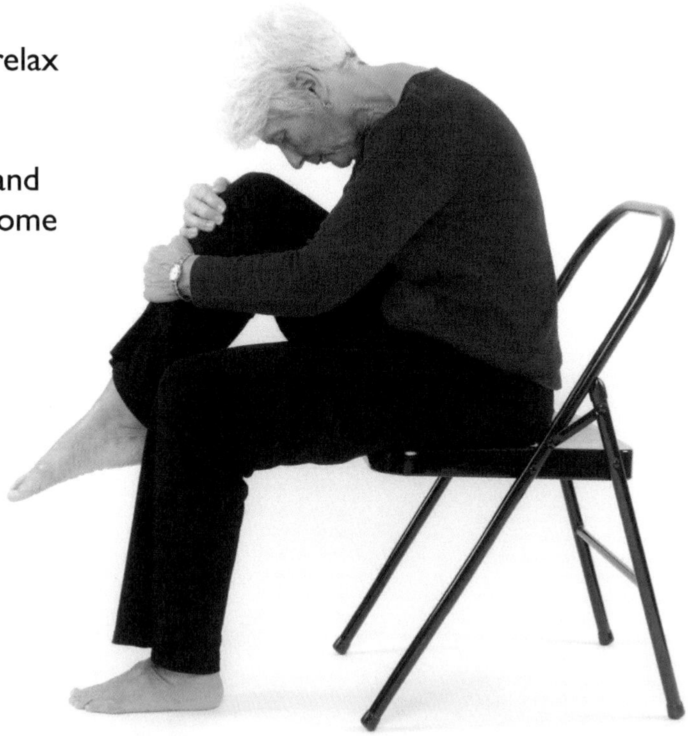

Half Inversion

Relaxes nervous system

Rest arms on legs reaching hands forward shoulder-width apart. Reach hands towards the floor. Hold and breathe.

Allow your head to hang. Keep chin tucked towards chest, tilt pelvis (navel up), and slowly come back up to sitting position. Lift head last.

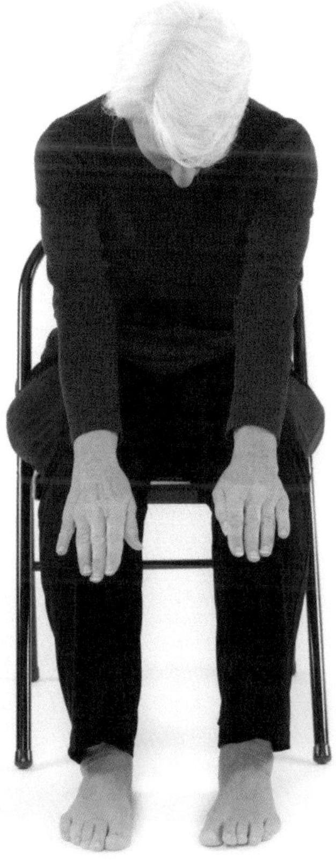

Cat

Lubricates the spine

Hands on thighs, seat, or seat sides of chair, pull shoulder blades down, lift tailbone, lift chest, look up, lift face towards ceiling (don't drop head back) keep back of neck long. Release hands and arms and relax them forward. Slowly bring chin to chest, round back, press navel to spine to curl the spine.

Repeat one vertebra at a time.

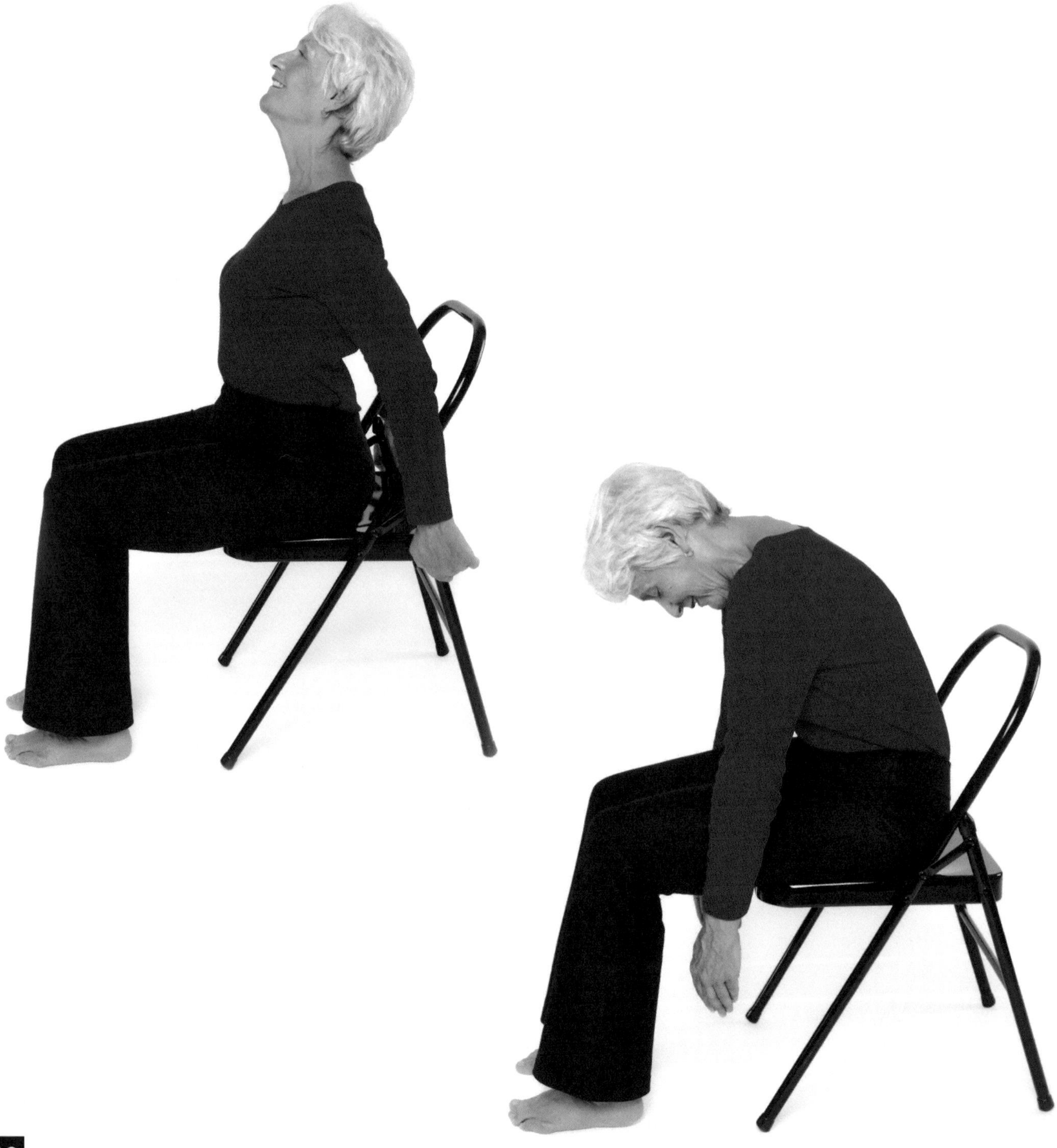

The following 5 poses are all lateral moves: Fan Palm, Half Moon, Dancer, Half Gate and Full Gate. It is not necessary to do every pose in every class as long as you take the spine in every direction. These are options to add variety to the Sit N Fit Chair Yoga program. Pick one (or more if you prefer) per class.

Fan Palm

Opens the ribcage muscles

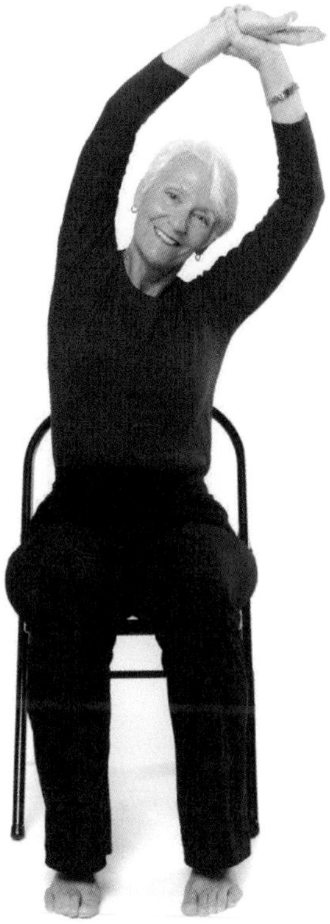

Right palm of hand up towards sky, fingers pointing towards left, hold right wrist with left hand, gently pull right wrist up and towards left. Press right shoulder slightly back to keep shoulder in line with right hip.

Repeat on left side.

Half Moon

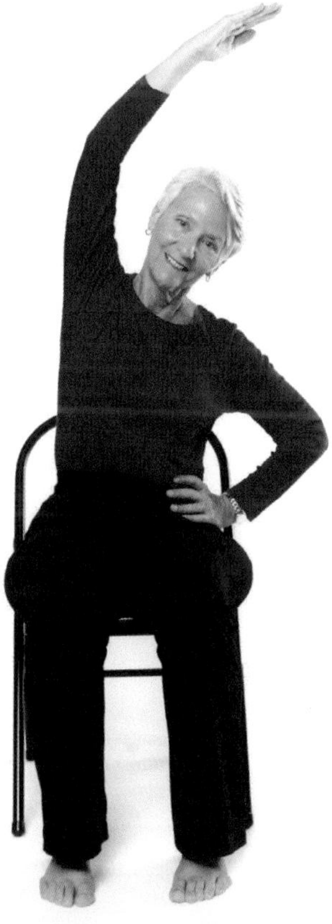

Slims the waist and stretches the sides

Left hand on left hip, right hand up and arm towards ear, palm towards head, right shoulder presses back to keep in line with right hip, tilt towards left, reverse.

Dancer

Stretches the sides

Touch left hand outside of left leg (towards calf or ankle), reach right hand up toward ceiling, look up or straight ahead, repeat other side.

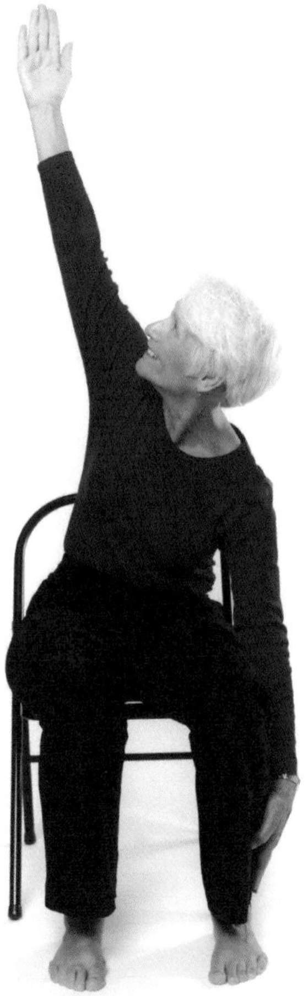

Half Gate

Opens the hips and stretches the sides

Turn right knee and foot out to right, bring right hand to right knee, left hand up towards ceiling, then towards right, keep shoulders in line with hips.

Repeat other side.

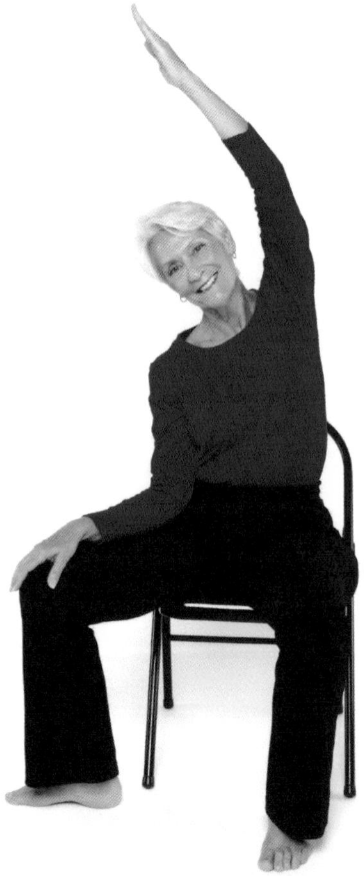

Full Gate

For more challenge extend left leg out to left, straighten knee, flex foot. Turn left palm up on left leg and slide hand toward knee or calf, keep shoulders in line with hips, reach right hand up towards ceiling, turn palm towards head, and bring arm towards ear.
Repeat other side.

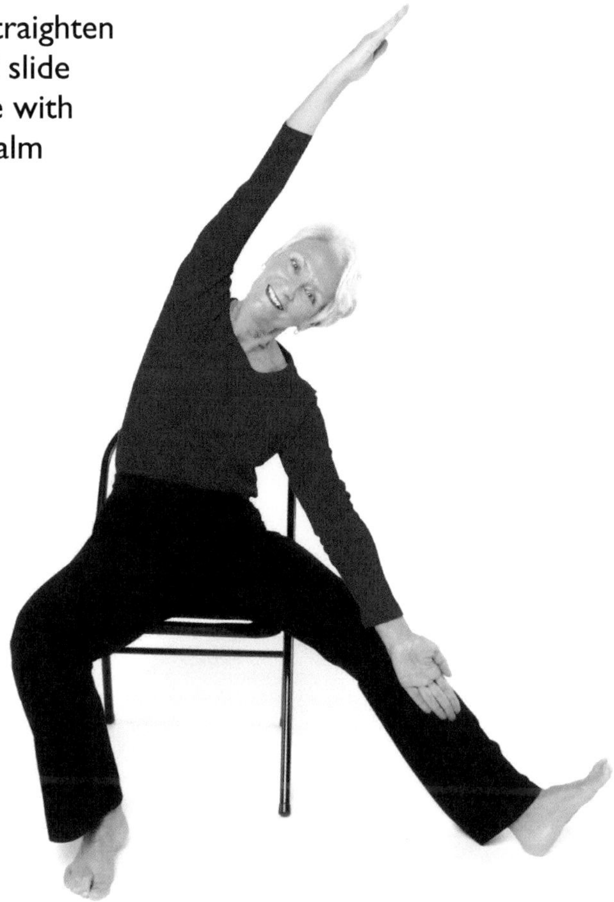

Sciatica Stretch

Stretches the muscles in the hips and back

Cross ankles or legs at knees, or ankle on knee (advanced), sit tall, hinge forward from hips. Hands and arms shoulder width apart rest on legs. Reach hands towards floor. Hold and breath. To come out keep chin tucked towards chest, tilt pelvis (navel up), and slowly come up. Repeat other side by reversing the crossed ankles, knees or ankle on knee.

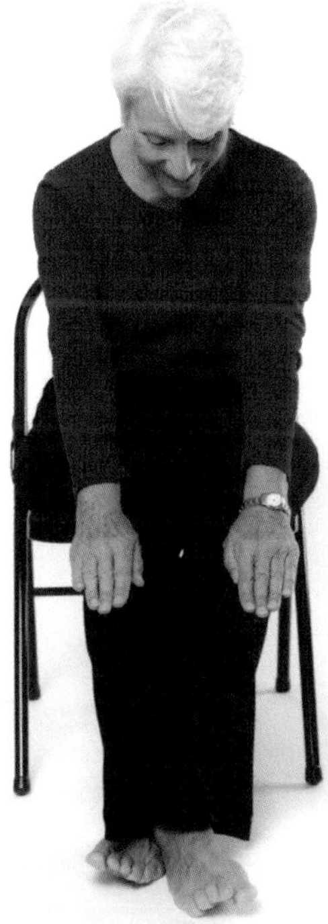

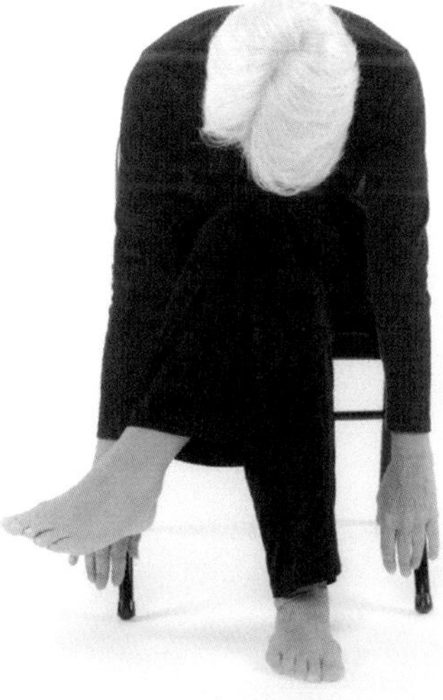

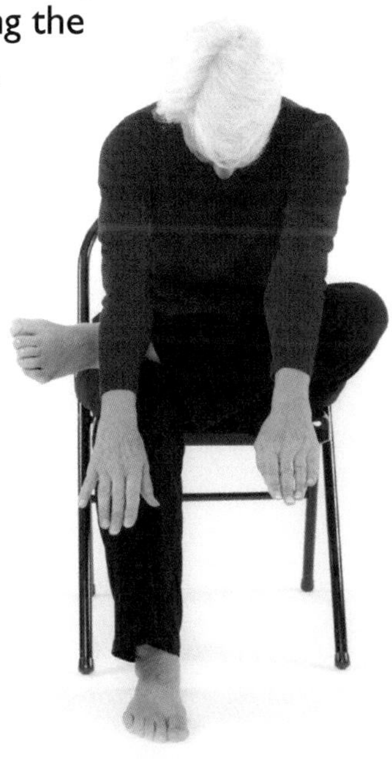

Seated Warrior I

Strengthens the legs, core, arms and shoulders

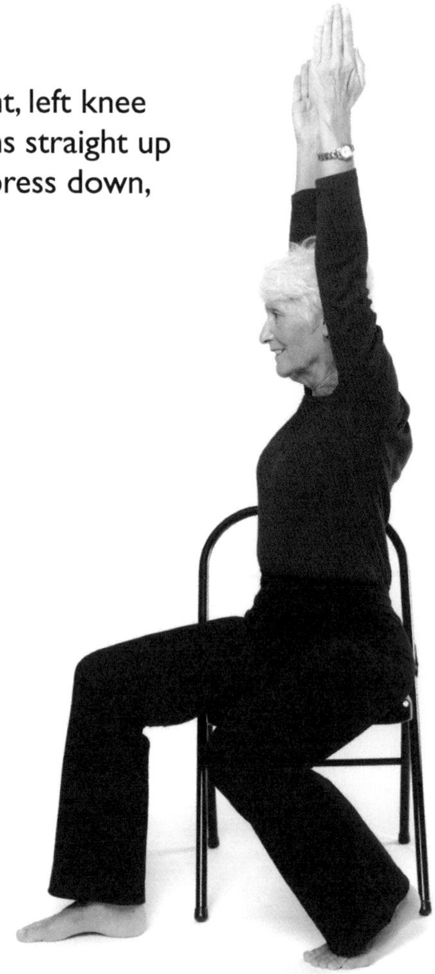

Step right foot out towards right, turn left foot right, left knee relaxes in, hands on hips, turn torso right, raise arms straight up from shoulders, palm facing palm, shoulder blades press down, look forward.

Repeat other side.

Seated Warrior II

Benefits include:

- *Opens the hips*
- *Strengthens the core, arms, shoulders and legs*
- *Opens the back muscles*

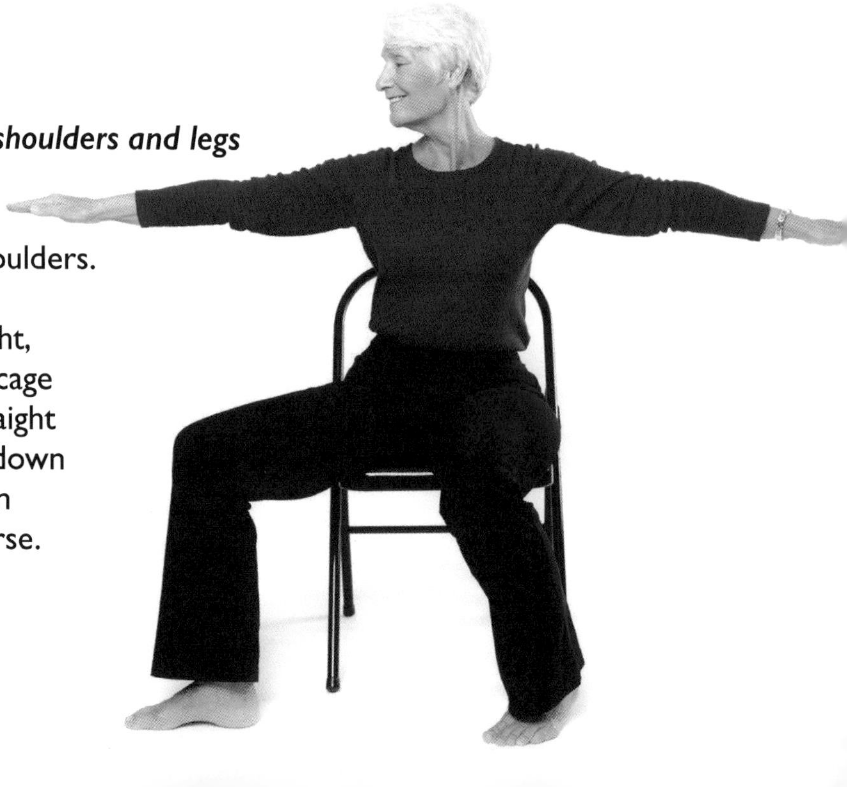

Legs wide, hips remain in line with shoulders.

Turn right toes right, left toes turn right, left knee relaxes towards right, lift ribcage and chest, raise arms in T position straight out from shoulders, lower shoulders down away from ears. Palms face down, turn head and look over right fingers, reverse.

Seated Cobra

Benefits include:

- ***Expands chest correcting rounded shoulders***
- ***Strengthens back muscles***
- ***Lubricates the spine***

Hands on thighs or seat sides of chair, pull shoulder blades down, lift chest, look up, lift face towards ceiling, keep the back of the neck long.

Slowly drop chin towards chest, tilt pelvis, round spine forward to come out and for a reverse stretch. Come back to a tall seated position.

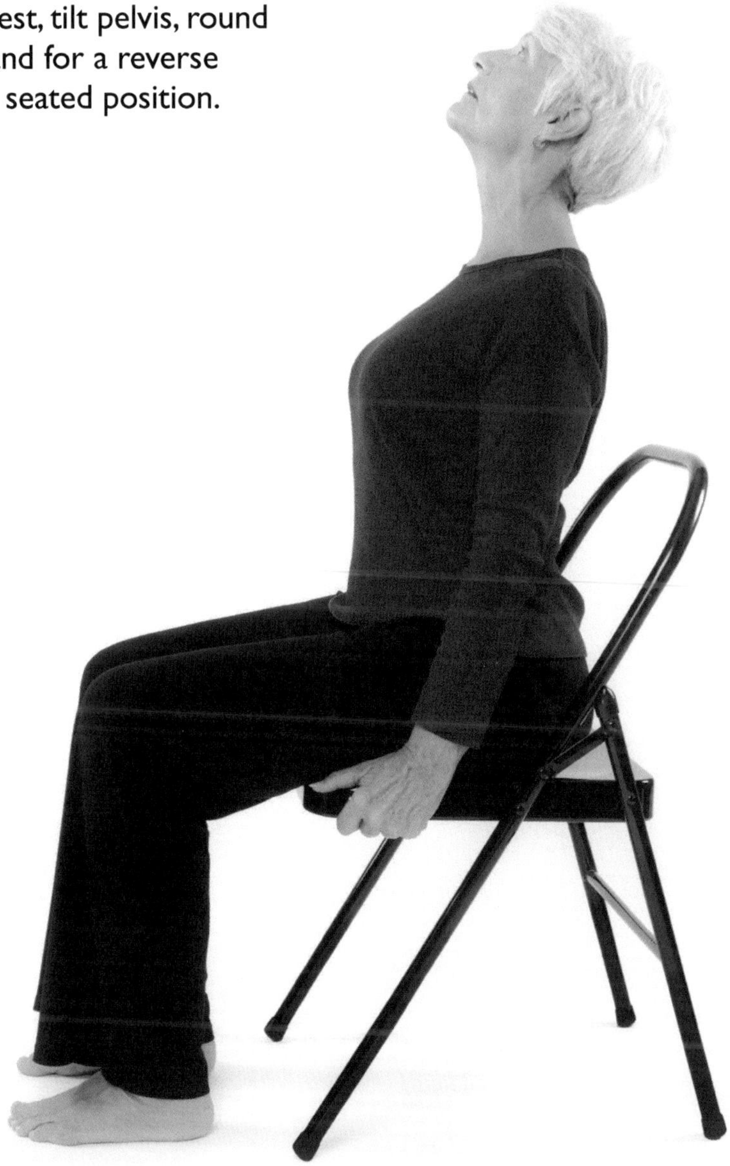

strong and open

Part 3: The Re-chargers

WARRIOR IN THE BODY Standing Poses – 5 to 10 minutes

If standing poses are not appropriate, go directly to Part 4, The Transformers, Mind Body Connection.

As students' progress, the following poses are done standing (holding the chair if necessary). The standing poses can replace the identical seated poses. Students may also continue seated. It is not necessary to do every pose in every class. It is recommended that the spine be taken in every direction in every class.

BALANCE

Mountain

Benefits include:

- *Strengthens ankles, knees and hips*
- *Corrects posture and strengthens core*

Feet hip-width apart, tuck buttocks slightly, lift ribcage, sternum, shoulders down, crown of head lifting, chin relaxed towards throat.

Knees are soft and not locked. Imagine a zipper located in the muscles between your legs. Squeeze and pull up the pelvic floor muscles as you zip up the imaginary zipper.

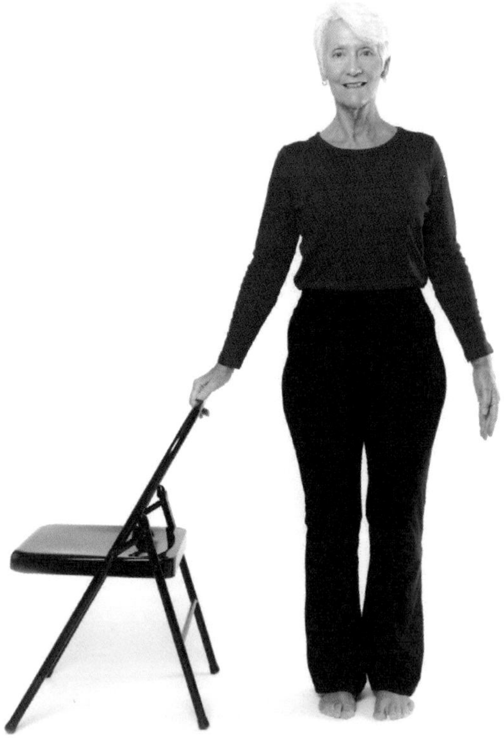

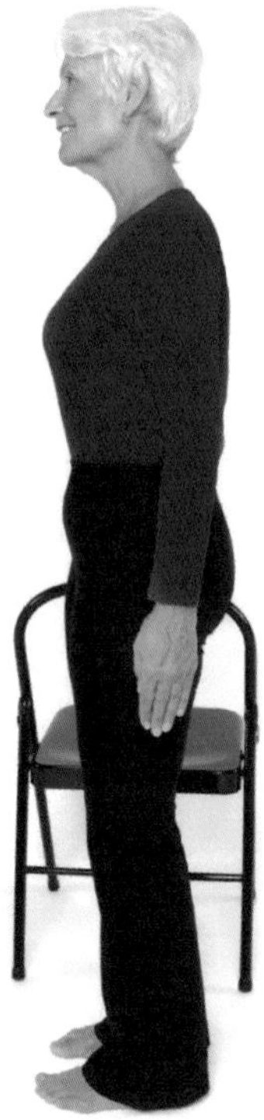

Stork

Strengthens stabilizing muscles and increases bone density

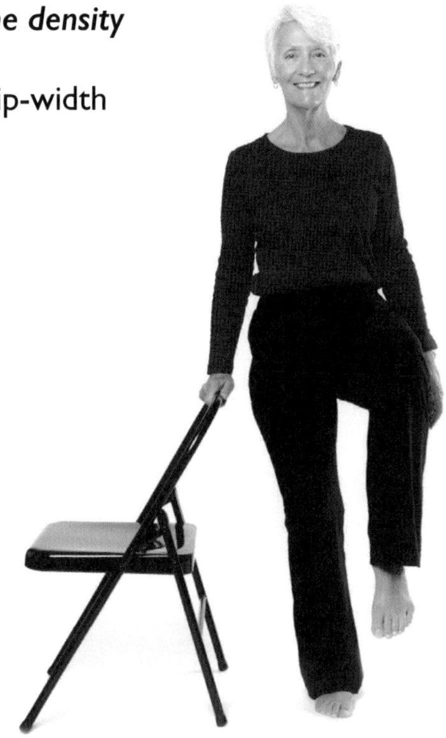

Focus eyes on a spot on the floor or wall. Feet hip-width apart or together.

Press weight into right foot, lift the left knee. Balance on one leg. Reverse.

Tree

Benefits include:

- *Tones and strengthens legs and core*
- *Opens the hip (if knee is turned out)*

Straighten spine with feet together or hip-width apart and press weight into right foot.

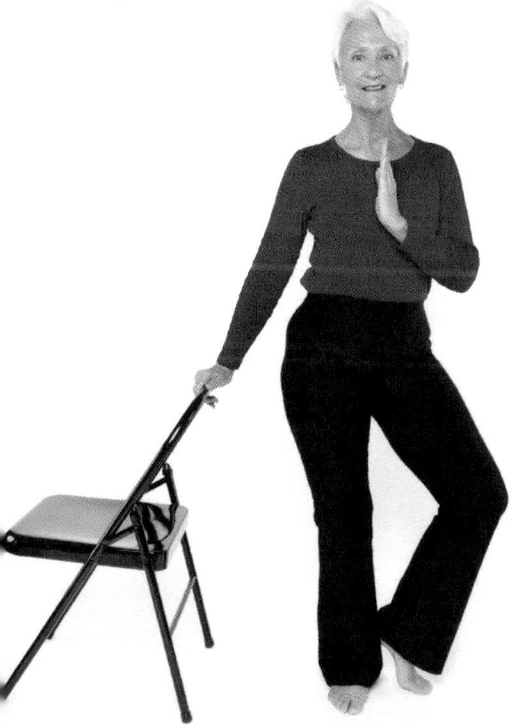

Bring left heel to right ankle, left knee pointing out to the left (or modify with knee straight ahead), or, for more advanced, heel to inside of calf, or thigh.

If holding the chair with right hand, bring left hand to the heart or above the head. Lengthen the spine. Hold and breathe. Reverse.

Advanced: palms together over heart or above head.

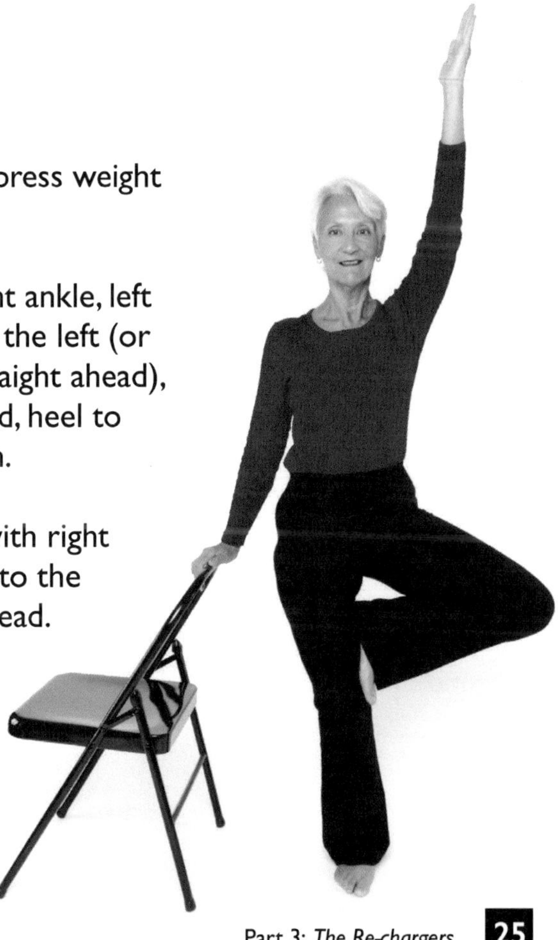

STRENGTHENING

Warrior I

Tones the whole body

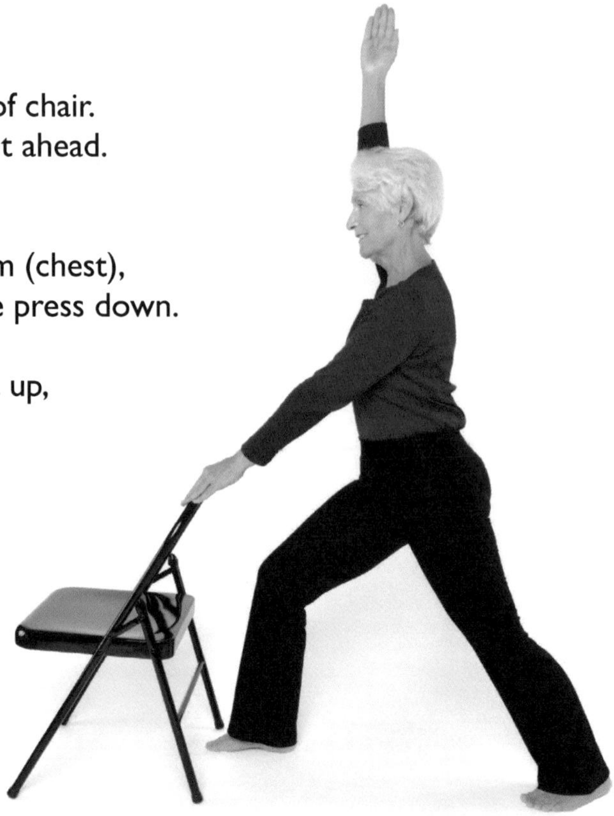

Stand behind back of chair and hold onto back of chair.
Step back with left foot, hips are squared straight ahead.
Legs and feet are in line with hips.

Bend right knee over ankle. Lift ribcage, sternum (chest), and crown of head, shoulder blades and tailbone press down.

Hold chair with left hand. Lift right arm straight up, palm facing head. Look forward.

To come out, lower arm, step left foot forward.

Repeat other side.

Warrior II

Tones the whole body and opens the hips

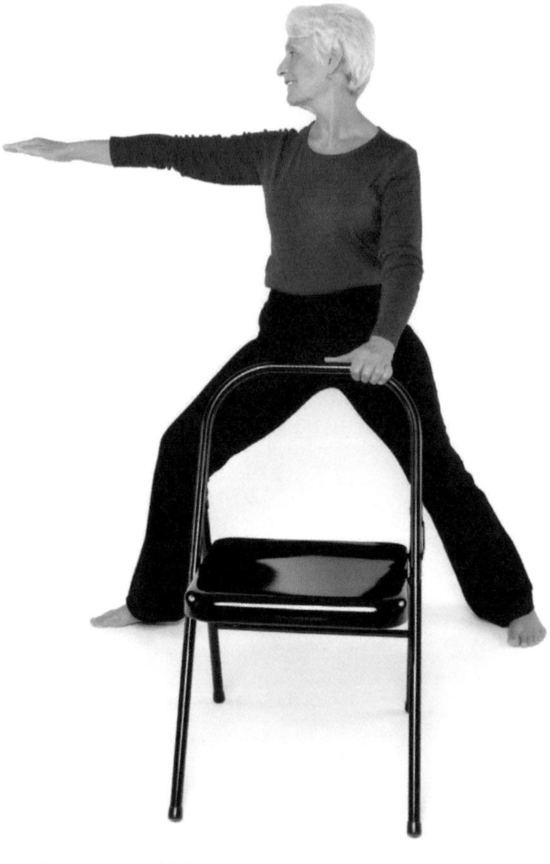

Stand behind chair, feet in line with hips, and hold back of chair. Step feet wide apart.

Torso and hips face chair.

Turn right toes right, left toes slightly in towards right. Lift right arm up shoulder height, palm facing floor, relax shoulders down, turn head slowly towards right.
To come out, lower right arm, hold chair.
Turn feet forward and bring feet back behind chair.

Repeat other side.

FLEXIBILITY

Half Moon

Benefits include:

- *Expands lung capacity and opens ribcage*
- *Slims hips and thighs*
- *Tones the legs*

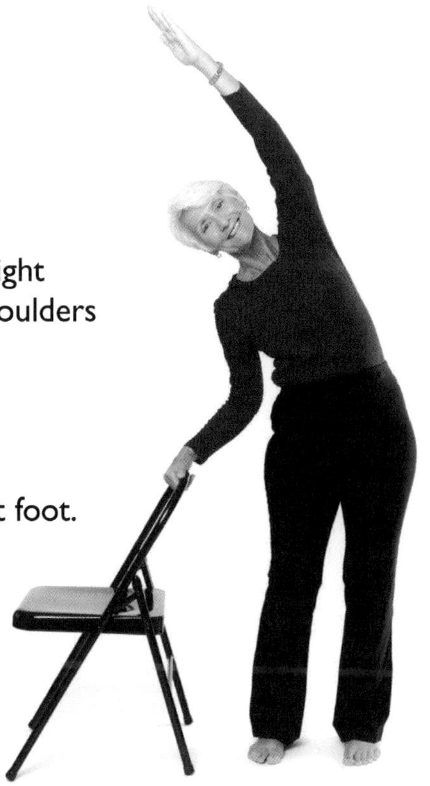

Feet hip-width apart. Holding back of the chair with the right hand, inhale the left hand up, palm towards head. Relax shoulders down away from ears.

Press into both feet and keep shoulders in line with hips.

Reach up and to the right with left hand and press into left foot.

To come out, straighten spine, lower left arm.

Repeat other side.

Triangle

Benefits include:

- *Promotes flexibility of hips and spine*
- *Tones body and legs*

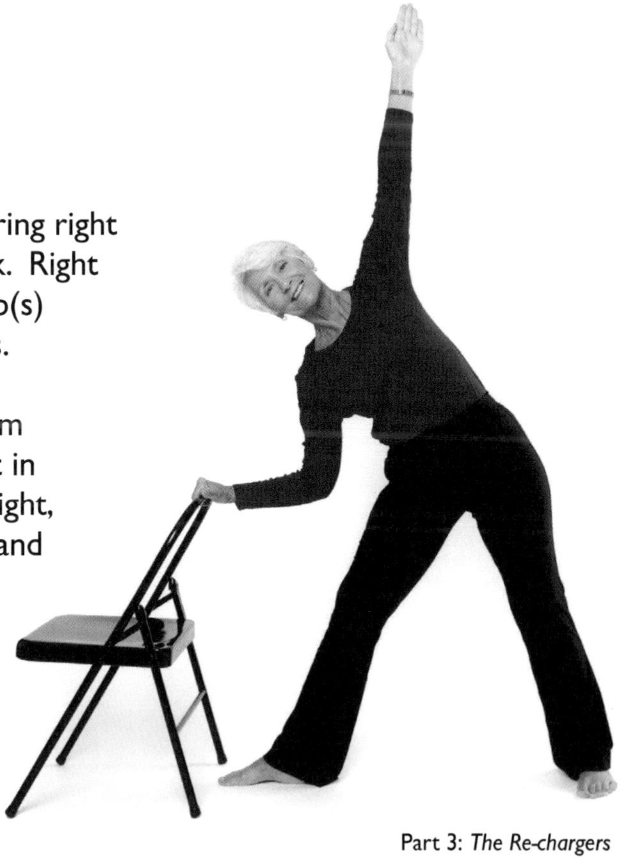

Stand behind the chair. Feet hip-width apart. Bring right foot towards center of chair. Step left foot back. Right toes point right. Both hands or one hand on hip(s) turn torso left. Bring shoulders in line with hips.

Straighten both legs if possible. Arms or one arm (if holding the chair) up shoulder height and out in a T position. Reach right hand and arm to the right, take left hip slightly to the left, and place right hand on chair back or seat. Reach left hand straight up from the shoulder (or left hand on left hip to modify).

To come out, lower left arm, turn torso and left foot to face chair and step back to the back of the chair. Reverse.

Advanced Triangle

Benefits include:

- *Promotes flexibility of hips and spine*
- *Tones body and legs*

Keep shoulders in line with hips, both arms and legs straight and look forward or up.

Stand behind the chair. Feet hip-width apart. Bring right foot towards center of chair. Step left foot back. Right toes point right. Both hands or one hand on hip(s) turn torso left. Bring shoulders in line with hips.

Straighten both legs if possible. Arms or one arm (if holding the chair) up shoulder height and out in a T position. Reach right hand and arm to the right, take left hip slightly to the left, and place right hand on chair back or seat. Straighten right arm. Reach left hand straight up from the shoulder (or left hand on left hip to modify). Look up or forward.

To come out, lower left arm, turn torso and left foot to face chair and step back to the back of the chair. Reverse.

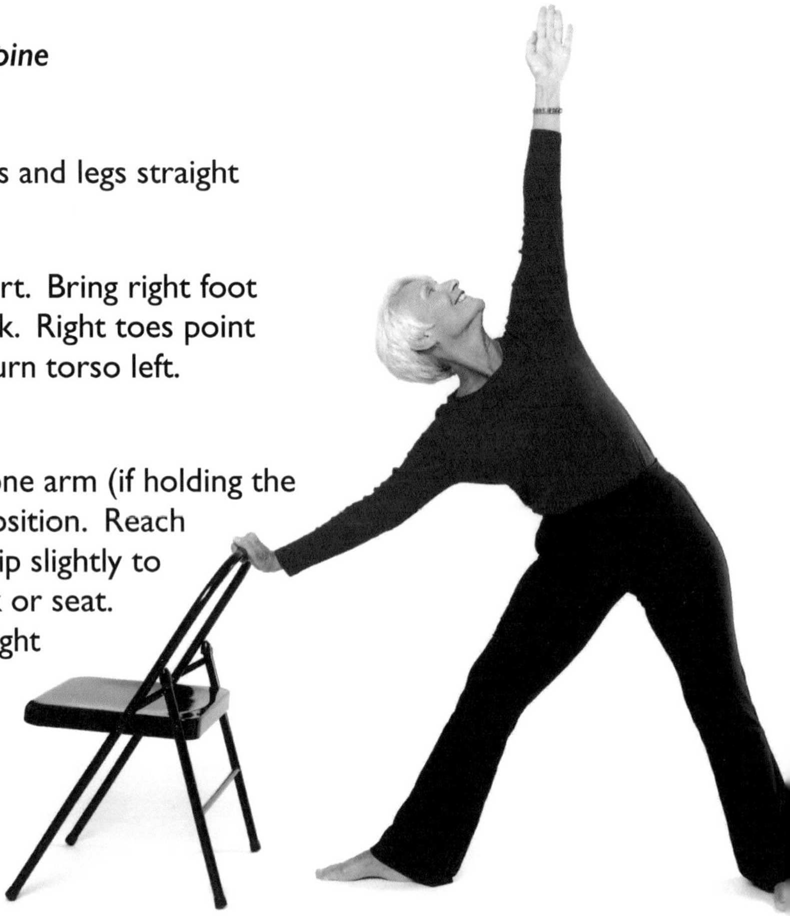

Cobra

Benefits include:

- *Creates length in the spine*
- *Opens the chest and ribcage*
- *Strengthens back muscles*

Holding back of chair, press into both feet, squeeze buttocks tight to protect low back, lift the ribcage and chest, draw the shoulder blades down, squeeze the shoulder blades towards each other and lift the face toward the ceiling.

Keep the back of the neck long.

To come out, relax the buttocks, tilt the pelvis (tailbone down, navel up) relax the shoulders, slowly bring the chin towards the chest then let the head return to a neutral position and look forward.

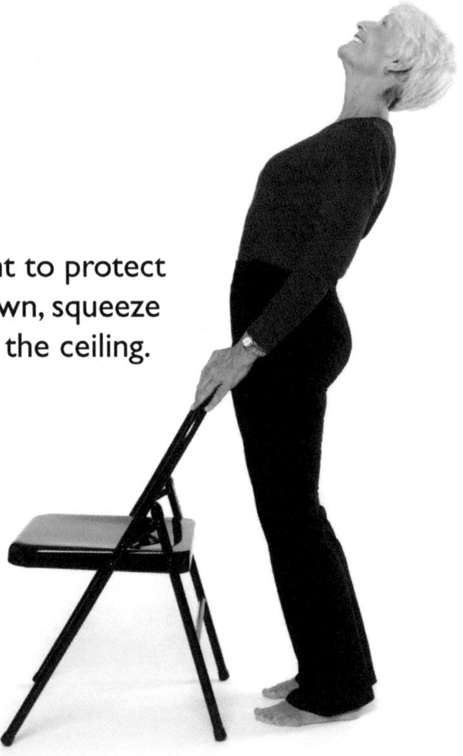

Locust

Strengthens the hamstrings, buttocks and low back muscles

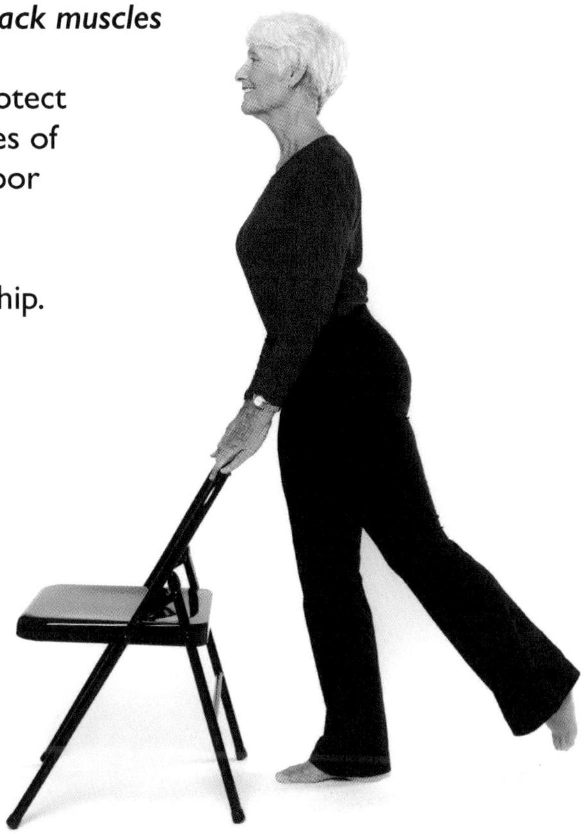

Hold back of chair, squeeze buttocks tight to protect low back. Press into the right foot. Take the toes of the left foot back, leave the toes touching the floor or lift the foot and leg.

To come out, return left foot and leg under left hip.

Repeat other side.

Table

Benefits include:

- *Stretches the back and hamstrings*
- *Lengthens the spine*

Hold the back of the chair, step back making a right angle with the arms and legs.

Bring the head between the arms and gently press the tailbone away from the head bringing traction and length into the spine.

To come out, slowly step forward towards the chair coming into a standing position.

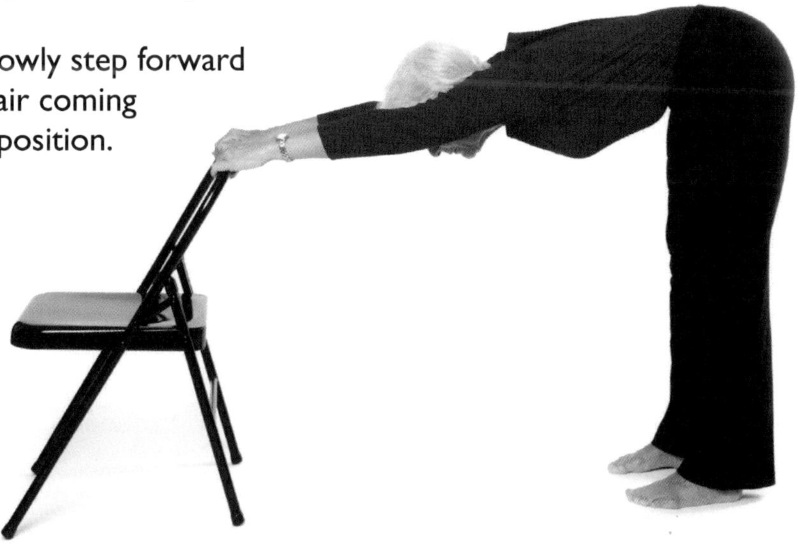

Part 4: The Transformers

MIND BODY CONNECTION – 10 to 15 minutes

Our cells have memory and as we go through our everyday lives, stress can be stored in the cells. Increasing body awareness will help you notice when you are feeling stress, i.e., tightness in the neck and shoulders. With this body awareness and practice, you will be able to neutralize and release stress. You will also know what your body is calling for. Maybe you need rest, water or oxygen. In the past, you may have always gone for food (sweets) not knowing what you really needed in the present moment.

Tense and Relax

Benefits include:

- *Tenses and relaxes one area of the body at a time*
- *Teaches body awareness*
- *Releases stress and tension*

Sit with a straight, tall, spine. Knees in line with hips. Hands relaxed on thighs or lap. Slowly begin to tense your right foot and leg. Squeeze it tight, tight, tight. Lift it up an inch or so, squeeze it tighter, tighter, tighter. Exhaling drop it. Relax it, let it go.

Slowly begin to tense your left foot and leg. Squeeze it tight, tight, tight. Lift it up an inch or so, squeeze it tighter, tighter, tighter. Exhaling drop it. Relax it, let it go.

Bring your attention to your abdomen. Pull your navel in, squeeze your buttocks tight. Hold that. Let go. Make fists with your hands, squeeze your arm muscles, pull your shoulder blades down, lift your chest up. Hold that tight. Release. Tense your neck by pulling your head down towards your shoulders. Release. Tense your face by scrunching it up. Let go. Slowly turn your head to the right as far as it will go. Slowly bring your head back to the center. Slowly turn your head to the left as far as it will go. Slowly bring your head back to the center. Bring your chin to your chest. Let your head go back to a relaxed neutral position.

Take a deep breath and exhale. Inhale again and tense your entire body. Feet, legs, abdomen, buttocks, hands, arms, chest, shoulders, neck, face, hold it tight! And release! Feel all of the tension leaving your body. The body and mind are quiet and still. You are serene and peaceful.

relax relax relax

Total-body Relaxation

Guided relaxation from toes to head

Sit with a straight spine. Rest the backs of your hands on your thighs, or palms up on your lap, right palm on top of left. Take a deep breath and exhale. Take another breath and let it go. Bring your attention to your toes and relax each one. Relax the soles of your feet and the tops of your feet. Relax your feet completely. Feel the relaxation coming into your ankles, relaxing your ankles, and then relaxing your shins and your calves. Relax your knees and all the muscles around your knees. Relax your thighs and hamstrings, the backs of your thighs. Relax your hips and your hip joints. Relax them completely.

Relax your fingers and thumbs. Feel the relaxation coming into the palms of your hands and backs of your hands. Relax your wrists, your forearms and upper arms. Relax your shoulders. Just let the tension melt away. Relax your abdomen. Relax all the muscles and organs in your abdomen. Let them melt down. Relax your pelvis, and relax your low back. Relax your ribcage. The front of your ribs and the back of your ribs. Relax your chest, your heart, and all the area around your heart. Release any holding around your heart and let your heart open. Relax your lungs. Let your breath be slow and gentle. Relax your middle back. Relax your shoulders again; relax them completely. Relax your upper back. Allow the chair to hold you.

Relax your neck, your throat and your jaw. Relax any tightness in your jaw or teeth. Relax your tongue, the back of your tongue and the muscles at the back of your throat. Let go of any unspoken words. Relax your face, all the skin and all the muscles in your face. Relax your temples and your ears. Feel the strands of tension release. Relax your eyes; just let them sink. Relax your forehead, your scalp, your hair follicles, and relax the back of your neck.

Relax your entire body. Feel your body in complete relaxation and remember what this feels like.

Forget the past, it's over. Let go of anything that no longer serves you.

Feel the peace. Just feel it. Drink it in and let it permeate every cell of your being. This is your true nature.

feel the peace

Visualizations

A transformed You! (use 1)

Guided visualizations of regenerated health

1. Visualize a brilliant white light at the crown of your head. Now see this healing white light gently spread to every cell and every atom in your mind and body. Every cell is now filled with light and love. Every cell is renewing and regenerating. You are refreshed, revived, invigorated and energized. Like a garden being nourished by the warm sunlight, refreshed by a gentle rain shower, fed by the rich nutrients of the earth, you draw in all the elements you need and you are transformed.

   You love yourself and take care of yourself every moment of every day.

   Intuitively you know just what to do. You are at peace.

2. Visualize a brilliant white light entering the crown of your head. Inhale the white light; filling every cell with energy, vitality, and life. Exhale a gray mist; releasing and letting go of any negativity. Inhale the white light; it will intuitively fill any cells calling for healing. Exhale the gray mist; let go of fear.

   I see my cells nourished.

   I see myself, healthy, whole, well and complete.

   I am at peace.

3. Deep, deep, deep at the core of your being is a peace so invincible no one can disturb it. No one can take this peace away from you. This peace is so powerful and unlimited, it is unending liberation from all suffering. In this peace is truth, light, and love. This is your true nature. Draw this peace into every cell of your being and know that it will intuitively go to any areas calling for healing.

   You are whole and nothing less than love . . .

   Remember who you are.

om shanti shanti shanti

References

1. Park J, McCaffrey R. "Chair Yoga Benefits for Community-Dwelling Older Adults with Osteoarthritis" Journal Of Gerontological Nursing Vol. 38 No. 5, 2012, 13-24

2. Park J, McCaffrey R. "The Effect of Sit N Fit Chair Yoga Among Community Dwelling Older Adults with Osteoarthritis" Holistic Nursing Practice – LWW Journals, Vol. 28 No. 4 2014, 247-257

3. McCaffrey R, Park J, "The Effect of Sit N Fit Chair Yoga in Older Adults with Moderate and Severe Alzheimer's Disease" Research in Gerontological Nursing, Vol. 7 No. 4 2014, 171-177

To purchase Sit N Fit Chair Yoga books and Sit N Fit Relaxation CD contact:

Email: *info@sitnfitchairyoga.com*
Website: *www.sitnfitchairyoga.com*

For mail orders:
Sit N Fit Chair Yoga
PO Box 7361
Delray Beach, FL 33482

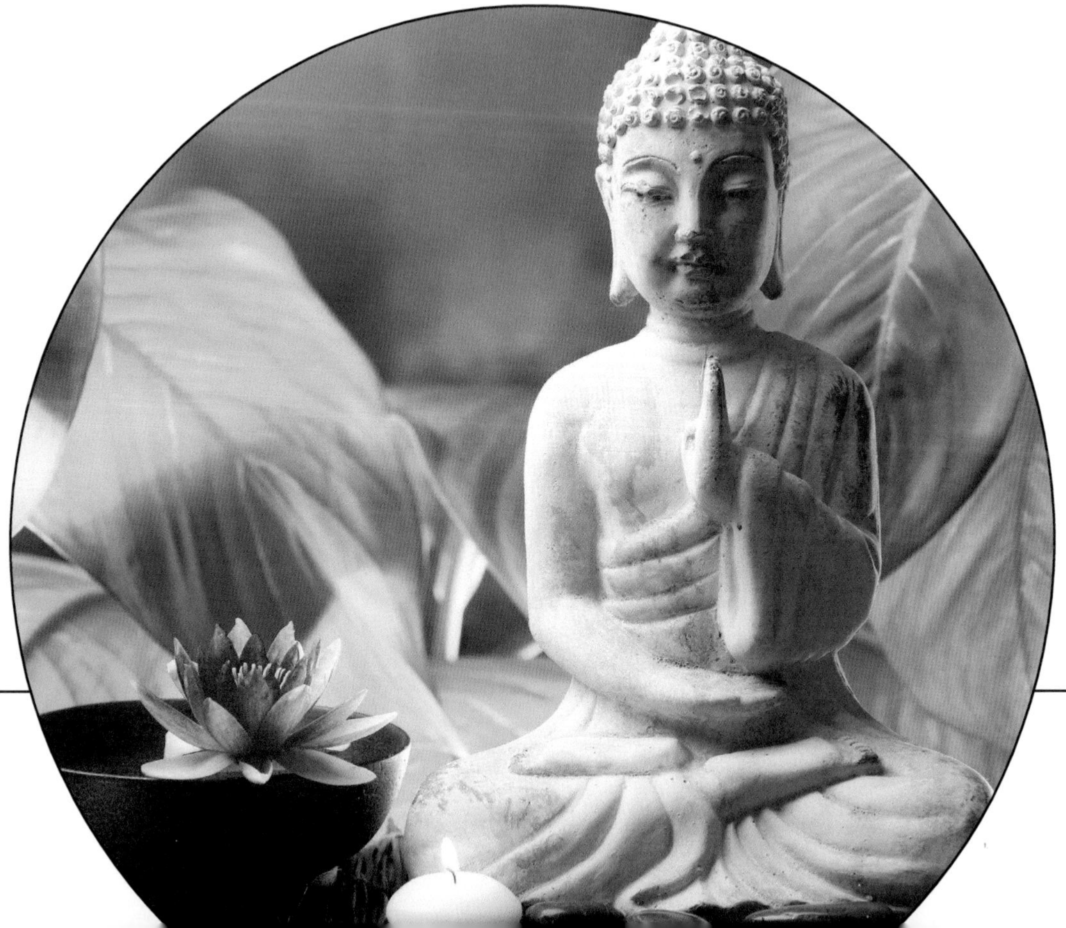

Printed in Great Britain
by Amazon

66194829R00026